A companion to the
overseas nurses programme

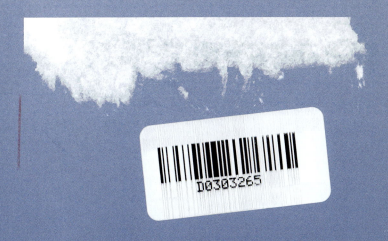

A companion to the
overseas
nurses
programme

Edited by

Jackie Hulse
University of Hertfordshire

PEARSON
Education

Harlow, England • London • New York • Boston • San Francisco • Toronto
Sydney • Tokyo • Singapore • Hong Kong • Seoul • Taipei • New Delhi
Cape Town • Madrid • Mexico City • Amsterdam • Munich • Paris • Milan

Pearson Education Limited
Edinburgh Gate
Harlow
Essex CM20 2JE
England

and Associated Companies throughout the world

Visit us on the World Wide Web at:
www.pearsoned.co.uk

First published 2008
© Pearson Education Limited 2008

ISBN: 978-0-13-238639-5

British Library Cataloguing-in-Publication Data
A catalogue record for this book is available from the British Library

10 9 8 7 6 5 4 3 2 1
11 10 09 08 07

Typeset in 9/13 Interstate Light by 3
Printed in Great Britain by Henry Ling Ltd, at the Dorset Press, Dorchester, Dorset

The publisher's policy is to use paper manufactured from sustainable forests.

Contents

Contributors

Note: At the time of writing, all contributors were in Nursing and Midwifery at the University of Hertfordshire with the exception of Ms Adris-Gilbert and Ms Beck.

Theo Adris-Gilbert
Lecturer, English Language Teaching Group

Siegrid Beck
Lecturer, English Language Teaching Group

Jane Clapham
Senior Lecturer

Christine Gault
Senior Lecturer

Kim Goode
Senior Lecturer

Jackie Hulse
Senior Lecturer

David Maher
Senior Lecturer

Ian Peate
Associate Head of School, Professional Academic Development

Philomena Shaughnessy
Associate Head of School, Practice Development and Enhancement

Foreword

As a member of the worldwide nursing community, you may now be considering a career in the UK. There are strong traditions within British nursing and to many these reflect the profession's roots. As you will know, the work of Florence Nightingale during the Crimean War was the beginning of modern nursing across the world. Nowadays in nearly every country the nurse is part of a profession regulated by law. To join the UK profession you may need to follow a course at a UK university that builds upon your existing professional expertise. This will ensure that you are well prepared to meet the exciting challenges that Britain has to offer.

Working within a Faculty of Health and Human Sciences in a UK University I have had strong links with the nursing profession over a number of years. Although I am not a nurse, I have appreciated the academic challenges of the transition of training for the profession as it moved into university-based education. The development of a multidisciplinary foundation for nurse education has enabled individuals to meet the range and scope of nursing practice, and to continue learning after qualification in order to meet future professional demands. Nursing is this nation's largest healthcare profession and individuals practise in a wide range of settings, from hospitals to GP surgeries to patients' homes. Their role is always developing, yet always remains central to the patient experience.

Teachers in the School of Nursing and Midwifery here have been working with overseas nurses for many years, and I am delighted to support the publication of this book, which is one of the first to be dedicated to the Overseas Nurses Programme. If you decide upon a career in the UK, I hope you enjoy the educational preparation that you follow and that the experience is the foundation for your continued professional development in whatever area of nursing you choose. Without doubt your professional qualification will always be in demand.

Dr Barry Hunt
Dean, Faculty of Health & Human Sciences
University of Hertfordshire

Introduction

Jackie Hulse

Welcome!

Welcome to this book on the Overseas Nurses Programme (ONP)!

You may have secured, or wish to secure, a place on the course. We hope that this book will be your guide to the programme, as well as helping you progress once you start your studies! Think of it as your 'workbook' and have your pen or pencil ready to start as you begin reading. In the book, there are some techniques designed to make your work and studies here easier, as well as plenty of exercises and activities to help you towards success. It will provide you with information that will be your guide through the ONP, and also help you to become aware of the responsibilities that both you and your employers have as you begin working.

Training for overseas nurses used to be called 'Adaptation' and you may still occasionally hear this term used, although it is no longer the official title. As an overseas nurse, you do not need to learn new physiology, and may not need to learn new medicines and techniques, but you do need to learn how to 'adapt' what you already know to how health care is delivered here in the UK. So the book begins with a chapter on **Reflection and Reflective Writing** which encourages you to explore your own skills and knowledge and consider how you may use reflective practice as a tool for success on the ONP.

The second chapter looks at the ever-changing **Role of the Nurse in the UK**, and is intended to allow you to consider your expectations and to appreciate how your previous role may differ. It also gives you an in-depth look at the Nursing and Midwifery Council (NMC) competencies. You'll be able to use your reflective skills here to determine your learning needs.

Finally, do remember that the ONP is about valuing your wide and interesting nursing experience, and helping you to focus and transfer your expertise to a UK setting.

GOOD LUCK!

Buchan J (2003). Nurse migration and international recruitment. *Nursing Inquiry* **8(4)**: 203-205.

Goodman B (2005). Overseas recruitment and migration. *Nursing Management* **12(8)**: 32-37.

Publisher's acknowledgements

We are grateful to the following for permission to reproduce copyright material:

Figure 1.1 from *Learning by Doing: A Guide to Teaching and Learning Methods* (Gibbs, G. 1988) with permission from Graham Gibbs.

The Nursing and Midwifery Council for extracts from: *The NMC code of professional conduct: standards for conduct, performance and ethics* (2004), http://www.nmc-uk.org and *Standards to support learning and assessment in practice: NMC standards for mentors, practice teachers and teachers;* The International Council of Nurses for *The ICN Definition of Nursing* (http://www.icn.ch/definition.htm) © 2006 by ICN.

Photographs
Alamy Images: Andrew Fox p. 92; David R Frazier Photolibrary, Inc. p. 95 (top); Geoff A Howard p. 93; Art Directors and TRIP photo Library: Helene Rogers p. 94; John Birdsall Social Issues Photo Library: pp. 87, 88, 90; Corbis: p. 96; Rex Features: p. 95 (bottom).

Picture Research by: Hilary Luckcock

In some instances we have been unable to trace the owners of copyright material, and we would appreciate any information that would enable us to do so.

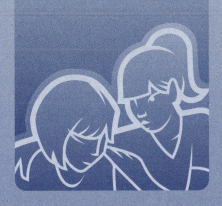

Chapter 1

How can I get the best out of my overseas nurses' programme?

Christine Gault

The aim of this chapter is to provide an introduction to the role of reflection and reflective writing as a tool for learning, documenting and improving practice. It will enable you to:

✔ Identify the purpose of reflective practice in professional life
✔ Consider why we emphasise reflection as a tool for nurses on this programme particularly
✔ Look at definitions of reflection
✔ Discuss some prominent theories and frameworks for reflection
✔ Identify how you can develop your skills as a 'reflective practitioner'

Nursing in the United Kingdom (UK) is a dynamic profession which strives to manage the changing health care needs of our society. One of the roles of the nurse is to meet the needs of the individual and society; therefore he/she needs to develop his/her theoretical knowledge continually, and support this by research and best available evidence. Additionally, the nurse needs to build on and expand his/her skills within the framework of professional practice. The standards and framework required of the nurse are published by the regulatory body, the Nursing and Midwifery Council (NMC 2004). It is particularly important for you as an overseas registered nurse, as we want to value and utilise your previous experience as you become accustomed to nursing in the UK.

Nurse education is committed to lifelong learning, widening participation, transferable skills and fitness to practise, as well as the ever increasing need for evidence of learning, e.g. the completion and production of a professional portfolio. There are a variety of learning strategies which can support the nurse as a lifelong learner; however, reflection is the most recognised as it encompasses a holistic approach to learning. Johns (2002) states that reflection involves all the senses to know our 'self' rather than a mere cognitive process. The NMC (2005) has advocated the development of the 'reflective nurse practitioner' by embedding reflection in the NMC's standards for post-registration education and practice (PREP).

It is essential that you acknowledge the nursing skills, knowledge and expertise that you have achieved as these will influence the quality of your future learning. These skills and knowledge are transferable within a variety of health care settings. However, perhaps the most important aspect is 'experience' as this combines knowledge and skills and applies them to practice. Benner (2001) suggests that experience provides the expert nurse with an intuitive grasp of situations, allowing them to identify the source of the problem. It is this experience which forms the basis on which reflection can take place.

It is not possible in a chapter of this size to cover all theories or frameworks for reflection; however, an introduction will be provided regarding the process as well as the basis on which you can start to use reflection as an active learning tool. Included is a toolbox of activities to support your reflection. Some activities are better completed with a partner or small group, others can be completed alone. You may wish to discuss issues arising as a result of the activities with a partner or mentor. There is no time limit set to completing activities; do them at your own pace and at a time that suits you.

What is the purpose of reflection?

The purpose of reflection is to examine and evaluate personal or professional experience.

Reflection is a window through which the practitioner can view and focus self within the context of her own lived experiences in ways that enable her to confront, understand and work towards resolving the contradictions within her practice between what is desirable and actual practice. Through the conflict of contradiction, the commitment to realise desirable work and understanding why things are as they are, the practitioner is empowered to take more appropriate action in future situations (Johns 2000, p. 34)

The aim is to gain insight, learn, develop and, when appropriate, change behaviour to enhance professional practice. It can support learning in the following areas:

- Self-awareness
- Personal learning
- Clinical practice
- Professional beliefs and values

Self-awareness relates to the extent to which we are conscious of our behaviour, emotions and how we relate to other people. Our unique 'self' has been shaped by our past, including cultural, social, emotional and spiritual factors. If behaviour is left unexamined then we may be unaware of the barriers we create in communication with others. When anxious or worried one may hide behind a façade of indifference or irritation, or we may appear assertive or aggressive when unsure or frightened. We may project anger onto others rather than acknowledge it as our own. It is through identifying our patterns of behaviour that we are able to develop a better understanding of ourselves. This is important as we need self-awareness to develop therapeutic relationships and work within a team or group (Bulman and Schutz, 2004).

Through reflection you can observe aspects of your behaviour and establish patterns emerging. Through evaluating situations you may be able to identify how you are presenting yourself to others. Self-awareness can assist in your personal learning.

To achieve the skills, knowledge and attitudes which are 'fit for practice' it follows that clinical experience is a fundamental component of your programme. Clinical work-related placements and the myriad of clinical experiences that come with them have many positive and enjoyable aspects associated with them; for example, an understanding of team roles and strategies for team working, learning from others in the team, and an awareness of the roles played by other professionals in health and social care in the UK.

Through the dilemmas and incidents on which you reflect, you will be able to identify and establish your personal philosophies, and how your culture, spiritual beliefs and experience of life have cultivated these philosophies. Often one can have a code of behaviour or belief system which has not been fully explored. It is only when applied to a situation or experience that these beliefs can be examined. For example, one may believe that all patients should be treated with respect but find this challenging when faced with a patient who is aggressive or abusive. Through exploring, debating and evaluating these issues within a framework of reflection, a professional or personal belief system can be established, producing a transparent and honest approach to our professional development.

 ## What about confidentiality?

You have a duty to ensure that you have maintained confidentiality in respect to all materials, including personal journals. You will need to bear this in mind as you begin to develop your reflective skills. Below is an excerpt from the NCM Code of Conduct (2004), which clearly identifies the nurse's role in maintaining confidentiality. Registrants have a duty to protect confidential information. Clause 5 of the Code is explicit in summarising what is expected of all registrants:

5.1 You must treat information about patients and clients as confidential and use it only for the purposes for which it was given. As it is impractical to obtain consent every time you need to share information with others, you should ensure that patients and clients understand that some information may be made available to other members of the team involved in the delivery of care. You must guard against breaches of confidentiality by protecting information from improper disclosure at all times.

5.2 You should seek patients' and clients' wishes regarding the sharing of information with their family and others. When a patient or client is considered incapable of giving permission, you should consult relevant colleagues.

5.3 If you are required to disclose information outside the team that will have personal consequences for patients or clients, you must obtain their consent. If the patient or client withholds consent, or if consent cannot be obtained for whatever reason, disclosures may be made only where:
   1. **they can be justified in the public interest (usually where disclosure is essential to protect the patient or client or someone else from the risk of significant harm);**
   2. **they are required by law or by order of a court.**

5.4 Where there is an issue of child protection, you must act at all times in accordance with national and local policies. *(Source: Nursing and Midwifery Council 2004)*

To trust another person with private and personal information is a significant matter. The patient/client has a right to believe that information given to a registrant in confidence is only used for the purposes for which it was given and will not be disclosed to others without permission.

Are there theories of reflection?

Dewey (1933), one of the earliest theorists on reflection, identified two modes of thinking. One mode was routine or habitual, such as the riding of a bicycle or cooking a meal; the second was reflection, which involves evaluating what you have done, why you did it and the outcome.

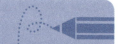

Activity

Habitual thinking: identify and list procedures in your professional practice which you perform in habitual or routine mode. How many are there? Take a few moments to make a list.

Dewey believed that reflective thinking was a natural response to a situation that the mind found difficult or perplexing. Reflection was, according to Dewey, nature's way to settle conflicting thought by searching for explanation or evidence. In a sense, the mind tries to find a meaning for something it does not understand.

There are several reflective models to help us do this and it is beneficial to explore and examine some of these to find a model which sits comfortably with your individual needs. The purpose of this section of the chapter is to demonstrate how you can use reflection as a learning tool. To do this we will use two frameworks.

Gibbs' framework for reflective thinking

The first framework is from Gibbs (1988) (Figure 1.1).

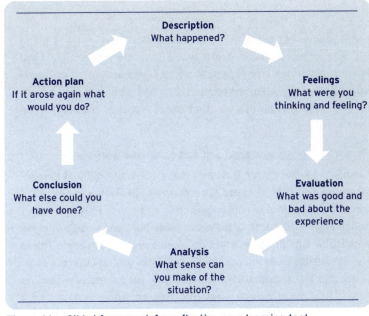

Figure 1.1 *Gibbs' framework for reflection as a learning tool*

The following reflective account demonstrates how Gibbs' cycle may be used as a reflective framework. It surrounds an incident when Nurse Scott has been asked to assess a new patient, Mrs Patel.

Description–what happened?

I was asked to assess Mrs Patel, who had just been transferred from the emergency department. She was breathless and receiving oxygen via a mask. I assessed her vital signs and recorded them. I asked her if she had any pain. She nodded her head to indicate 'no'. I went to retrieve her notes. When I came back Nurse Harris was sitting by her bed holding Mrs Patel's hand and gently talking to her. Mrs Patel was crying. Nurse Harris asked to see Mrs Patel's treatment chart to assess her prescription for pain relief as Mrs Patel said she had pain in her chest and her back.

Feelings—what were you thinking and feeling?

I was annoyed at being asked to assess Mrs Patel as I was going off duty in half an hour and it would take me longer than that. When I saw Nurse Harris with Mrs Patel I immediately felt inadequate and angry. I had asked her if she had pain; why did she not tell me she did? I always feel that Nurse Harris is checking up on me.

Evaluation—what was good and bad about the experience?

I realised I knew better than to behave the way I did and demonstrate my feelings of anger towards my patient. It was not that I was being unkind or unprofessional with Mrs Patel. I wasn't behaving in a deliberately dismissive way but I just wasn't thinking about how I might be presenting myself. Having observed Nurse Harris I realise I was unconsciously telling Mrs Patel I was too busy. Nurse Harris demonstrated how to use your eyes and ears to listen. It showed me an empathic side to Nurse Harris that I had not seen before. I have always been jealous of her efficient way.

Analysis—what sense can you make of the situation?

My feelings of jealousy and exasperation got in the way of me using my skills in identifying Mrs Patel's pain.

Action plan—if this situation arose again, what would you do?

I need to be aware of my feelings and the impact they have on my behaviour. The next time I feel angry or annoyed, be aware and think about what I am doing and feeling.

The framework is arranged in a cycle, as the action plan should then change your behaviour if you were in a similar situation again.

Let us look at the framework when used by Nurse Harris given the same incident.

Description—what happened?

I was administering my drug round when I came to Mrs Patel, a new patient. She looked so anxious and distressed that I locked the drug trolley and sat next to her. After introducing myself, I asked her if she had any pain. She nodded 'no' but I wasn't sure, as it was difficult to see her expression with the oxygen mask on. I took her hand and made eye contact. She was crying and, when I asked if she had pain, she nodded yes. She said she had pain in her back and chest which was worse when she breathed in. I stayed for a few minutes until her nurse came back and suggested she review Mrs Patel's pain relief.

Feelings—what were you thinking and feeling?

I felt sorry for Mrs Patel; she looked so vulnerable and afraid. I was aware that I did not want to be distracted from the drug round but I could not have ignored her.

Evaluation—what was good and bad about the experience?

I guess it was good that I stopped what I was doing to help Mrs Patel. It was a pity I did not have more time to spend with her.

Analysis—what sense can you make of the situation?

I realise I can get caught up in routine and tasks. It would have been easy to ignore her but that's not what I am there for. Her nurse was obviously busy.

Conclusion—what else could have been done?

I could have stayed and helped Mrs Patel's nurse make her more comfortable. I could also liaise with the emergency department about patients being sent to the ward without pain relief. We do not always have the drugs in stock. I must talk to the ward manager about this.

Action plan—if this situation arose again, what would you do?

Go with my instinct when I think someone is in pain.

Nurse Scott recognised that her emotions were overshadowing her behaviour. Interestingly, she assumed that Nurse Harris was thinking she was not good at her work. Yet, in Nurse Harris's account there was no mention of this. Bolton (2005) suggests that no-one can **know** what really happened in any situation but can express their understanding and perception of what happened. It is this understanding and perception, in the forefront of the nurse's mind, that needs to be explored and expressed.

Often we are not aware of how other people perceive us. It would be easy simply to ask what they thought of us, but how honest would they be? Perhaps the best measure of how we appear to others is through their behaviour or reactions towards us.

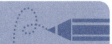

Activity

Learning from reflection: identify and discuss how the reflective accounts given by Nurse Scott and Nurse Harris may have contributed to their learning in the following areas:

- Self-awareness
- Personal learning
- Clinical practice
- Professional beliefs and values

Rogers (1961) identified congruence, empathy and unconditional positive regard as a basis for developing a therapeutic relationship. Being unable to be genuine in how we express our feelings, or not understanding the other person's view of the situation, or being judgemental can create barriers to effective communication. According to Thompson (2002), self-awareness can develop confidence in ourselves and others. As we recognise the impact our behaviour has on others we can become aware of how other peoples' actions and attitudes impact on us. Thompson (2002) also suggests that self-awareness is important in dealing with prejudice, discrimination and oppression within society.

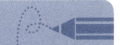

Activity

Identify a situation when you recognised that someone had the wrong impression of you, or of something you had done. Write a description of the situation. Observe how you are feeling, your emotions and reactions as you write.

- When was the defining moment that you realised they had the wrong impression of you?
- What may have led to this perceived difference?

Model for structured reflection (Johns 2000)

This model may be a useful framework for a more complex detailed analysis. Johns (2000) supports the use of a structured diary, the idea being to bring experiences together to support greater learning. His framework reflects Carper's (1978) four patterns of knowing:

- Aesthetics
- Personal
- Ethics
- Empirics

Carper (1978) suggested that personal knowledge underpinned the therapeutic use of 'self'. Johns (2000) brings knowledge and therapeutic use of self together.

The first stage of the reflection framework is the preparation of time, environment and mind. Johns (2002) suggests this 'looking in' is similar to preparing to meditate. This is followed by 'looking out', giving a description of the experience followed by cues which help 'deconstruct' the experience to develop understanding which can then be applied to future experiences.

Aesthetics

What was I trying to achieve?
Why did I respond as I did?
What were the consequences of that for:

- *The patient*
- *Others*
- *Myself*

How was this person(s) feeling?
How did I know this?

I remember being in a hospital and being told that my grandmother had died. I was not thinking about this when I went to see Mrs Coley but I suddenly had an overwhelming feeling that I wanted to scream and so wanted to run out of the room but could not. I had to be 'professional'.

I guess I did run away when I was in the room. I focused my attention on the patients outside, rather than stay with Mrs Coley and her son. Mrs Coley and her son appeared shocked and confused. I could have been a supportive presence if I had stayed.

Personal

How did I feel in this situation?
What internal factors were influencing me?

I have always thought that I was really good with relatives and have always taken time to sit and listen, but in this situation I felt a panic that I did not expect. To be honest, I think there were two factors which made me react the way I did. Firstly, I did not know the relatives or Mr Coley; it was so sudden and I often feel uncertain of people I have not met before. I like to build up relationships as it makes me feel more secure – perhaps I was feeling vulnerable. The other factor was my grandmother's death. I have not been home since she died; I often forget she has died and then get a shock when I remember.

Ethics

How did my actions match my beliefs?
What factors made me act in an incongruent way?

Although I would like to think that my behaviour was not influenced by my emotions, in this situation it would not be true. I was unable to contain the situation or myself.

Empirics

What knowledge did or should have influenced me?

I have done a short course on breaking bad news. I understood it was important to have privacy, etc. In a sense I was restricted by the resources available. However, the knowledge did not prepare me for the emotion and panic I experienced in myself.

Reflexivity

How does this connect with previous experiences?
Could I have handled this better in similar situations?
What would have been the consequences of an alternative act for:

- *The patient*
- *Others*
- *Myself*

How do I now feel about this experience?
Can I support myself and others better as a consequence?
Has this changed my ways of knowing?

Having examined the situation in greater detail I feel less guilty. The main learning for me has been that, as nurses, we are all people with our own life experiences. I did not know that I held onto the death of my grandmother. I wonder what other issues might arise that I am unaware of at present. However, I do not believe that to be professional you need to be emotionless, but perhaps be able to contain one's emotions or at least not let them get in the way of your duty of care.

It also made me appreciate the support of the nursing team in the department. I spoke to a couple of nurses about how I was shocked by my reaction. They shared similar experiences that they had had with me and how they felt about it.

This experience has changed me; it has highlighted to me the importance of my self-awareness and has also made me more aware of my colleagues as emotional, feeling, professional people.

Reflective writing

Review your own behaviour as you have read this chapter. Several activities have asked you to take notes. If you did not take notes then ask yourself why not? It may be that note-taking is difficult or that you learn more by thinking or discussing. In one aspect of professional practice the NMC requires evidence of learning and also a record; record-keeping is a fundamental requirement of nursing practice.

If you did take notes you will have the notes to refer to later. By recording and writing, we reinforce learning and this provides greater insight. The process of writing provides structure but also gives another opportunity for analysis.

By keeping a record over a period of time you can look for themes in your work which reoccur and perhaps are not resolved, or conflicts that present themselves in a variety of forms. Casement (1990) recommends the use of your 'internal supervisor' as you write. This involves listening to your own thoughts and feelings as you write and including them in your account. It provides a safe base for you to explore your feelings. Hull *et al.* (2005) suggest that you may censor what you write if you are concerned about offending others. This might disrupt the process, so it is important to set some ground rules on how you are going to ensure you keep your record safe and secure.

The purpose of reflective writing is to support the process of reflection while, at the same time, providing evidence of learning. Aspects of your records may be required for teaching and learning or for your professional portfolio. It is up to you to decide which aspects are confidential and which aspects are not.

Keeping a journal

The key to journal-keeping is organising it in such a way that it suits your personal needs. The topics in your journal may include:

● Surprises or anxieties regarding your clinical practice

● Situations, incidents or experiences that resonate with you

● A record of your practice

● A demonstration of good or poor care

● A comment from a patient or relative

● Situations when you felt challenging emotions either from a patient, colleague or self

You can then use aspects of your journal for the purpose of reflection and a record of learning. Use whatever tools you prefer, such as a coloured pen, highlighter, diagrams or drawings. You may prefer to keep a journal electronically. Burns and Bulman (2000) suggest journals may be kept private and selected aspects can be used for reflective essays or profiles.

There are several methods that you can adopt to record your reflections. It is essential that you use one that best suits your learning style. If writing does not feel comfortable the chances are you will not do it and evidence will be lost both for your personal and professional development.

It is often difficult to find the time in practice to write a description of a situation. **Mind maps** can be helpful as they give you the opportunity to record the main themes when they are fresh in your mind and you are still clear on how you are feeling. You can then use them to describe your experience when you are in the correct environment and have time. This is demonstrated in Figure 1.2.

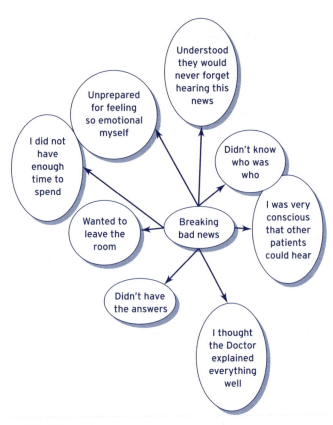

Figure 1.2 *Mind map*

Activity

Identify a situation or event from your professional practice.

Using a mind map identify all the aspects you need to consider.

Identify:

- best available evidence such as policies, protocols or relevant literature that might relate to your situation
- people involved and their contribution
- your thoughts and feelings at the time

It may be helpful to discuss this with a peer or mentor

Case Study

Scenario B

Nurse Baker has to renew Mrs Cohen's wound dressing.

It was a difficult afternoon; I had a headache and wanted to have my break early so I could have something to eat. Mrs Cohen required a renewal of her dressing and was to have her analgesia 20 minutes before the change of dressing so I needed to plan it well. I had never used this dressing before but Nurse Carty had offered to demonstrate it to me.

Nurse Carty said she would be free at 13.30 hrs so I was too late for first break and would need to go later. At 13.10 hrs I gave Mrs Cohen her analgesia and told her we would be back to change the dressing. I prepared the dressing trolley and went to find Nurse Carty. It was 13.20 hrs and she had just gone on her break and would be back at 13.50 hrs. I felt a surge of anger. We could have gone to coffee together and then done the dressing but now Mrs Cohen was ready and I w~~as not~~ ~~_____~~ ~~headache was__~~ getting worse. What should I do?

There was no-one free to help me. Should I call Nurse Carty back from her break . . . she will be angry. I could leave the dressing until the afternoon, but Mrs Cohen has had the analgesia and is ready. Besides, her son is visiting later in the afternoon. I wished I had watched this dressing last time it was done. Perhaps it will be OK to change the dressing when staff nurse returns . . . I just don't know.

Activity

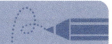

Identify a situation or event from your professional practice.

Use a reflective framework of your choice to explore the situation or event.

Discuss this activity with a peer or mentor.

You may wish to include this activity as part of your professional portfolio.

Developing the skills of reflection is a vital component of the overseas nursing programme (ONP). The knowledge, skills and experience you bring to the programme will provide the basis on which your learning can develop. Remember also that reflective writing is at the core of the portfolio that the NMC will require you to keep for periodic re-registration. The NMC (2005) has produced templates and examples of how reflection may be documented.

In order to expand your skills in reflection, a commitment to the following is required:

- A belief and willingness to change and develop your professional practice.
- Commitment to develop your self-awareness and identification of your strengths and limitations.
- Embarking on lifelong learning.

It is evident that learning through reflection is challenging, as the skills required involve evaluating personal beliefs and behaviour. A reflective framework can provide a focus and widen the scope on which to base these discoveries. This will allow you to learn and discover new dimensions of 'self' and professional practice and, in doing so, provide high quality and effective nursing care which can make a difference to your patients, society and profession.

Summary

This chapter has outlined:
✔ **The purpose of reflection.**
✔ **Theories and frameworks for reflection ... have you found a framework that you think will be useful for you?**
✔ **Examples of situations where reflection could help the nurse in everyday practice.**
✔ **Suggestions and exercises on how to get started as a 'reflective practitioner'.**

References

Benner P (2001). *From Novice to Expert : Excellence and Power in Clinical Nursing Practice. Commemorative Edition*. New Jersey: Prentice Hall Health.

Bolton G (2005). *Reflective Practice Writing and Professional Development*, 2nd edn. London: Sage.

Bulman C and Schutz S (2004). *Reflective Practice in Nursing*. Oxford: Blackwell.

Burns S and Bulman C (2000). *Reflective Practice in Nursing: The Growth of the Professional Practitioner*, 2nd edn. Oxford: Blackwell Science.

Carper B A (1978). Fundamental patterns of knowing in nursing. *Advances in Nursing Science*. **1(1)**: 13-23.

Casement P J (1990). *Further Learning from the Patient*. London: Tavistock Publications.

Dewey J (1933). *How We Think: a Restatement of the Relation of Reflective Thinking to the Educative Process*. Boston: Heath.

Gibbs G (1988). *Learning by Doing: A Guide to Teaching and Learning Methods*. Oxford Brookes University: Further Education Unit.

Hull C, Redfern L and Shuttleworth A (2005). *Profiles and Portfolios: A Guide for Health and Social Care*, 2nd edn. Hampshire: Palgrave Macmillan.

Johns C (2000). *Becoming a Reflective Practitioner: A Reflective and Holistic Approach to Clinical Nursing, Practice Development and Clinical Supervision*. London: Blackwell Science.

Johns C (2002). *Guided Reflection Advancing Practice*. Oxford: Blackwell Science.

Nursing and Midwifery Council (2004). *The NMC Code of Professional Conduct: Standards for Conduct, Performance and Ethics*. London: NMC.

Nursing and Midwifery Council (2005).*The PREP Handbook*. London: NMC.

Rogers C (1961). *On Becoming a Person*. London: Constable.

Thompson N (2002). *People Skills*, 2nd edn. Hampshire: Palgrave Macmillan.

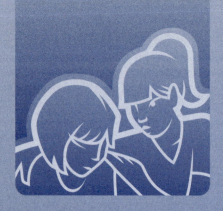

Chapter 2

The role of the nurse in the UK: meeting the competencies of the Overseas Nurses Programme

Jackie Hulse

This is a key chapter for you to read. It will help you to understand what you will be doing here as a 'learner' on the ONP. The chapter will enable you to:

✔ Identify the role of the NMC and professional self-regulation
✔ Discuss some professional conduct issues
✔ Explore the competencies established for the ONP
✔ Consider key differences in nursing practice that you might expect and thus
✔ Identify your own related learning needs and priorities

This chapter begins by assuming that you have a wealth of experience on which to draw and skills to offer, but that you may not know how nursing 'works' in the UK. As we will discuss later when looking at cultural issues, there is much that may be familiar to you and much that will be new. Rather than try and describe what a nurse does here, we will look at the competencies that the NMC have determined for the ONP, so that you can see quite clearly what is expected of you. Finally, the chapter will look at some of the issues which the NMC tells us can cause problems for nurses.

What is the role of the NMC?

The Nursing and Midwifery Council is an organisation set up by Parliament to protect the public by ensuring that nurses and midwives provide high standards of care to their patients and clients. To achieve its aims, the NMC has the following responsibilities: maintains a register of qualified nurses, midwives and specialist community public health nurses; sets standards for conduct, performance and ethics; provides advice for nurses and midwives; considers any allegations of misconduct, lack of competence or unfitness to practise due to ill-health.

http://www.nmc-uk.org/aSection. aspx?SectionID=5

Let us look at what this is telling us about your relationship with the NMC. Firstly, the NMC maintains the Register that you are hoping to join, and regulates the professional conduct of nurses and midwives, whatever their sphere of practice.

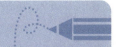

Activity

Are you familiar with professional self-regulation? How is nursing regulated at home? What challenges do you think self-regulation brings?

In order to regulate, the NMC must have a tool against which to measure and so sets standards and guidelines for practice. You can obtain these from the NMC website and are particularly advised to look carefully at the NMC Code of Professional Conduct: Standards for Conduct, Performance and Ethics. This may be quite similar to the standards you are used to, but you need to study it carefully to ensure you can practise according to its precepts. The NMC also provides advice for registrants on topics such as consent, advocacy and autonomy, and medicines management, to mention just a few from a huge list! This advisory service is intended to support nurses and midwives in providing effective and appropriate care at all times, and enabling them to be constantly aware of their responsibilities. Lastly, the NMC deals with conduct and competence issues. Before we look at competence and misconduct, do remember that the NMC is also responsible for looking at cases where the problem is due to ill-health rather than deliberate misconduct, and that the NMC will try to support registrants in such difficulties. However, the patient/client's interests will always come first and so we must all demonstrate that we are 'fit for purpose', i.e. mentally and physically well enough to nurse.

What does nursing mean to you?

You will probably have studied many different definitions of nursing during your initial nurse education and you may well have your own particular favourite. I like this, from the International Council of Nurses (ICN):

Nursing encompasses autonomous and collaborative care of individuals of all ages, families, groups and communities, sick or well and in all settings. Nursing includes the promotion of health, prevention of illness, and the care of ill, disabled and dying people. Advocacy, promotion of a safe environment, research, participation in shaping health policy and in patient and health systems management, and education are also key nursing roles.

www.icn.ch/definition/htm © 2006 by ICN

Does a definition of nursing and a search for shared values actually help you to understand the *role* of the nurse in any particular country? You may find that you have a lot in common in terms of shared values with your new colleagues but does that help you to identify and begin to examine their daily work and the extra skills and knowledge that you may need for it? The English dictionary defines a role as 'the typical or classical function performed by someone or something' (Oxford English Dictionary 1994), so we need to try to characterise that role for you so that you can start to identify your learning needs.

 ## What does the NMC expect of overseas nurses?

If you look on the NMC website or in an overseas information pack, you will find the competencies that they have devised, and I have listed them for you at the end of this chapter. Just as interesting as the competencies themselves are the headings or domains in which they are grouped. These are:

- Professional and ethical practice
- Care delivery
- Care management
- Personal and professional development

These headings tell us that the NMC is concerned that nurses are working with full awareness of professional and ethical imperatives, with an emphasis on *both* care delivery and care management. It has an expectation that nurses will be committed to lifelong learning and professional development. Let us take a closer look at some of the competencies and try and extract some of the challenges they may pose.

 ## What are the competencies for professional and ethical practice?

- Manage oneself, one's practice, and that of others, in accordance with the NMC's Code of professional conduct; standards for performance, conduct and ethics, recognising one's own abilities and limitations.

What does this suggest to you? What will be your immediate learning needs? I think that it means you will need to be familiar with the Code of Conduct for one thing, but it reminds us that we must only ever act within our competence. Imagine the scene ... a patient is in distress waiting to have a surgical drain removed ... you have never seen it done but are sure you could do it and, anyway, you are really upset that the patient is distressed. Have you ever been tempted in such a situation? What would be the correct course of action? Additionally, there may be aspects of care that you would be accustomed to performing at home (Allan and Larsen 2003; Gerrish and Griffith 2004), but which do not form part of the nursing role here. Thus, time spent observing and 'shadowing' the work of your mentor will be invaluable in helping you to explore the role of the nurse here. This competency also reminds us that, as registered nurses, we must manage the work of others. I would suggest that one of the first things to do, therefore, is to understand the work of other members of the team.

Activity

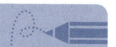

Take a look around at other members of the care team ... What are their roles? How do they differ from yours? What do you need to know about their work and how will you find out?

This is an important activity for you to think about ... don't assume that the roles you are used to will be the ones that are common here. For example, although called by different names, many countries have care assistants, but their roles and functions will not be the same. As a reg-istered nurse you are responsible for ensuring that individuals are not given tasks for which they are not competent. Conversely, nobody can take responsibility for *your* actions except *you*. If a colleague gives you an instruction that you don't understand or is outside your capabilities then, even if that colleague is a senior nurse or doctor, any actions taken remain your responsibility. This competency also reminds us of the need to be sure that colleagues are practising to high standards and are able to deal appropriately with any concerns. The thought of criticising colleagues may sound very awkward for you if you still feel like a 'visitor' here, but it is important to bear in mind that this is the cornerstone of professional self-regulation.

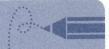
- Practise in accordance with an ethical and legal framework which ensures primacy of patient and client interest and respects confidentiality.
- Practise in a fair and anti-discriminatory way, acknowledging the differences in beliefs and cultural practices of individuals or groups.
- Demonstrate openness and acknowledge differences in between your own culture and that in a multicultural UK.
- Demonstrate knowledge of the ways in which health and social care is established and delivered in the UK.

What are the legal and ethical imperatives for nurses in the UK? A comprehensive and popular book on legal issues and nursing is that by Dimond (2005), but you might well find your own particular favourite. In the early pages Dimond reminds us that the nurse is accountable in four ways: to the criminal courts, to the civil courts, to professional bodies, and to an employer (p.10). This book clearly identifies the legal imperatives for nurses across a range of settings, and discusses the knowledge and decision-making skills that will help a nurse practise safely. Many of you will come from countries where the law and legal framework for care are very similar to those in operation here. However, that is not universally so, and thus it will be worth identifying key areas where laws may differ or be complex or even appear to you to be controversial. Caulfield (2002, p. 111) offers a salutary reminder in pointing out that 'only 20 years ago it would have been a struggle to find even one textbook that referred to the law and clinical practice. Now there are many books specialising in the area.' One point to stress immediately is that Scottish criminal law is, and always has been, distinct from the rest of the UK, and the Scottish Court of Appeal is still the final arbiter in criminal cases. Political devolution will also mean changes to how health law is made and interpreted in other member countries of the UK, which will inevitably impact on nursing practice there.

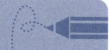

Activity

What do you think are key areas of law that nurses need to consider?

Caulfield (2002), Dimond (2005) and Fletcher and Buka (1999) all discuss issues relating to **consent**, **confidentiality** and **negligence** amongst general issues of importance. Caulfield also identifies particular laws relating to **euthanasia**, **termination of pregnancy** and **organ donation**, with which you may or may not be familiar. Do you recall that the NMC competency spoke of the 'primacy' of the patient? This principle is especially strong in UK health care, even if it may have surprising consequences. Caulfield relates the example of a patient in Broadmoor Hospital (a hospital for those with mental health problems ordered to be detained by the Criminal Courts) who refused an amputation for a gangrenous leg. Caulfield (p. 114) reports that 'the court agreed that his decision should be respected even if it meant that he could die without the treatment that was regarded as being in his best interests by the clinical team.' I would urge those of you working with children/young people and the elderly to be particularly vigilant about issues of consent and confidentiality, and recall your duty of care to the individual rather than to any family or carers.

If legal aspects are about keeping within the law, then how would you define ethical aspects? Fletcher and Buka (1999) suggest that ethics is a way of expressing moral rules and that society expects 'ethical behaviour on the part of health care professionals' (p. 162). But whose ethical code? Even more than legal frameworks, I would suggest that ethical codes are mediated by cultural norms. One interesting example is the priority or pre-eminence given to the individual in western societies that some would find unusual or unacceptable. Parker and Clare (2002, p. 221) reiterate four ethical principles for health care that you will find advocated generally in the UK:

- Autonomy: the right a person has to direct their own life and make their own decisions
- Beneficence: the responsibility of doing good
- Non-maleficence: the responsibility to avoid doing harm
- Justice: the responsibility to be fair in the way we treat others

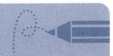

Activity

Can you think of a situation that posed an ethical dilemma? How did you resolve it?

The challenge for nurses is that we don't live or work in a perfect world where there is only ever one right answer. The NMC thus reminds us of the need to be able to demonstrate and justify the legal and ethical basis to our practice. If you are interested in this area of care, I would recommend any of the books mentioned, but you might also like to have a look at the challenging work of Seedhouse (2000, 2005) who is a Professor of Health and Social Ethics in New Zealand.

To meet these competencies you will also need to be familiar with cultural and social trends in the UK, and in particular where you are working. You can read more about this in Chapter 5. Do remember that culture is not just about the person. It may even affect the disease or problems that bring them into your care, and indeed how they respond to them (Spector 2004). Above all, though, I think that these competencies are asking you to take a look at your own values and beliefs, and consider where and how they may differ from those of your patients. True anti-discriminatory practice comes not from being free of prejudices or personal beliefs, but from keeping these personal feelings away from your practice and ensuring that you truly 'empower' your patients to make choices for health. Chapter 1 looked at how the skills of structured reflection may help you in difficult situations. Reflection on your previous practice, and whilst in practice with your mentor, will then further your development.

What about care delivery and management?

These represent the bulk of the competencies that have been set for you, and so we will go through and extract the sense of what they convey, rather than look at each one individually.

Activity

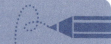

I have not listed them in the same order as they appear in NMC publications; I have grouped them together according to the 'themes' each one represents. Have a look at them and then decide on the themes that occur to you.

- Engage in, develop and disengage from therapeutic relationships through the use of appropriate communication and interpersonal skills.

- Undertake and document a comprehensive, systematic and accurate nursing assessment of the physical, psychological, social and spiritual needs of the patients, clients and communities.

- Formulate and document a plan of nursing care, where possible in partnership with patients, clients, their carers, and family and friends, within a framework of informed consent.

- Demonstrate sound clinical judgements across a range of differing professional and care delivery contexts.

- Based on the best available evidence, apply knowledge and an appropriate repertoire of skills indicative of safe nursing practice.

- Evaluate and document the outcomes of nursing and other interventions.

- Accurately interpret numerical data and their significance for the safe delivery of care.

- Accurately calculate and administer prescribed medication.

- Understand and follow complex lines of argument in a health care topic.

- Read and understand new knowledge from articles in nursing journals.
- Effectively interact with a degree of fluency and spontaneity that makes information sharing with patients/clients and their relatives and colleagues possible.
- Actively participate in discussions about health care and patient issues, accounting for and sustaining personal views.
- Effectively report in writing and verbally, passing on information or producing reasoned justifications for actions in different situations.
- Contribute to public protection by creating and maintaining a safe environment of care through the use of quality assurance and risk management strategies.

What themes have you identified? There is no ideal answer to this but, as a framework for looking at the competencies, I would suggest that we consider:

- **Assessment, planning, delivery and evaluation of care**
- **Acquisition of, and communication of, knowledge, both for patient care and professional development**
- **The nurse and quality assurance**

You are, without doubt, accustomed to using the nursing process to plan and deliver nursing care and probably to assess patients, set goals and determine outcomes. This is one of your greatest transferable skills ... every nurse should be able to assess a breathless patient and come to some decisions about nursing needs. Remember that you have not lost your observational skills! So where will the differences lie? Probably in the tools and the nursing language that you use (Hardill and Macdonald 2000) and the organisation of that care (Gerrish and Griffith 2004).

It would be impossible to explore every type of nursing care plan in such a short chapter and so I can do little more than emphasise that the application of the nursing process from assessment to evaluation remains one of the key and core skills for nurses whatever the setting. Your task will be to adjust or adapt your observations, assessments and care goals into the format and language that you find in use wherever you work. Chapter 6, on language skills and your growing reflective skills, will undoubtedly help you with this. The Department for Education and Skills (DfES 2005) has published some wonderful resources that you could work through, and these include exercises to help you become accustomed to the tools and language that we use. Studies mentioned have suggested that organisation of care is an area that may differ from what some nurses are expecting. 'All overseas nurses commented on the differences in the organisation of care. Many were more familiar with a more task-orientated approach' (Gerrish and Griffith 2004, p. 582).

Thus, it would be well worth having a look at some of the types of care delivery systems. Cronin and Rawlings-Anderson (2004) review these quite succinctly. The evolution from task allocation through patient allocation to **team nursing**, **primary nursing** and its **key worker** variants are all discussed. They point out that some of these systems, such as 'named nurse', were really products of the political climate of the time and are no longer promoted in government initiatives, but have evolved into other systems (p.138). You will find different care delivery models in operation in different settings, but it is likely that whatever system is in use, it will be patient-focused and aimed at continuity of care, and will involve nurses taking responsibility for the holistic care of individuals rather than performing tasks. Cronin and Rawlings-Anderson also point out that care delivery is constantly developing, as much as anything to keep pace with the changes in roles and service delivery models. There is every sign that this will continue as the drive for interprofessional working and seamless care continues.

Activity

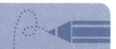

With what sort of care organisation are you familiar?

What are the advantages and disadvantages of different systems?

During the course of care planning and delivery, you will also be expected to demonstrate decision-making skills and an evidence base for those decisions. It is vital to realise that UK nursing prides itself on having an evidence base that can be independent of other professions. A good example of this is in the area of tissue viability, where nurses lead other professionals in research and the application of knowledge (Chambers 2002). Many of you will be accustomed to this role for the nurse, but some of you may come from health systems still dominated by doctors and the medical model (Crookes *et al.* 2002), and may find this particular exercise of accountability to be a challenge. Gerrish and Griffith (2004) do suggest that some overseas nurses have found the informality between nurses and between nurses and doctors rather unexpected, and that they did not feel comfortable 'challenging any decisions' made by senior nurses or doctors. The competencies also include the expectation that you will become familiar with drug administration here and be able to calculate drugs and fluids appropriately. The NMC regularly updates its guidelines on the administration of medicines, and you can expect to be introduced to the system in use in your placement during your orientation.

Activity

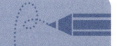

What do you think is meant above by 'Accurately interpret numerical data and their significance for the safe delivery of care?'

Linked to this, indeed an essential prerequisite, is the knowledge that forms the basis of care planning and care decisions. What is the nature of this knowledge?

I am sure that most of you have suggested that this will be the data generated by patient observations or discussions, and the competency expects you to be able to make an observation and decide on appropriate action. That action might involve recording and repeating the observation, reporting to a senior colleague, or calling for medical help. The skill is in making the right choice for that patient in that care setting at that time! This is when it is so important to take full advantage of your supernumerary learning time during the ONP. This is time you can spend with your mentor or another colleague and see how they handle these situations. Then remember to ask yourself, 'What would I have done had it been my decision?'

Where else does 'nursing knowledge' come from? The obvious answer is from research published in scholarly and professional journals, which is why it has been included in the competencies. Once again, you may be accustomed to browsing through such journals routinely and sharing information with colleagues. But if you are not, then this is an area upon which you will need to concentrate. You could try selecting either a topic of interest or one related to the speciality of the placement area and set yourself the task of finding relevant articles. You could then move on to deciding how to use them to inform your practice. The most important thing is to realise that this is in the ONP competencies because it is expected that every UK registered nurse is both conversant and comfortable with knowledge generation and retrieval. Once knowledge is generated, it then needs to be disseminated and evaluated, which is why communicating knowledge has been given such a priority. Student nurses here are taught that they must always understand the rationale for any care that they give, and that they should be able to discuss and justify it, which is really what is being asked of you.

I would suggest that there is another dimension to the competencies on communication as well, and that is the role of the nurse as care coordinator and patient advocate. Some overseas nurses have voiced surprise at the apparent contradictions in UK nursing, in which some technical roles are only carried out by nurses with special training (e.g. cannulation), but nurses are expected to be at the centre of coordinating a complex multidisciplinary discharge (Gerrish and Griffith 2004). Liaison with members of other disciplines involved in patient care and discharge planning for those patients will be a significant part of your role depending on the setting. You will also be expected to attend ward and care/case meetings to discuss patients' care and to contribute to the decisions made.

The last competency in this section concerns your roles in quality assurance and risk management activities. These two are central components of clinical governance (see Chapter 7), but it could be argued that nurses have always been concerned with quality. That does not mean that it has become any easier to measure, and remains enigmatic; as Jasper (2002, p. 402) says 'quality is a nebulous term that means different things to different people ... it is clearly meaningless to talk about quality care without defining the standard of quality that you are aiming for'. Clinical governance has introduced structures that are intended to make continuous quality monitoring improvement an integral part of health care delivery rather than an adjunct or specialist activity.

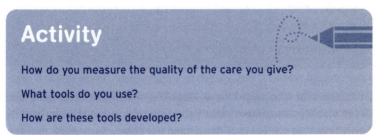

Activity

How do you measure the quality of the care you give?

What tools do you use?

How are these tools developed?

Thus National Service Frameworks (NSFs), together with Scottish Service and Welsh Service Frameworks, are available to provide 'clear, common, national standards for service provision' (Clayton 2003, p. 7). Much of the decision-making about what constitutes a reasonable standard will be influenced by the work of the National Institute for Clinical Excellence (NICE), which is the national body which appraises and advises on the suitability and sustainability of treatments. You will have noticed that this relates to service provision and not just nursing care, but NICE does have a nursing arm, the National Collaborating Centre for Nursing & Supportive Care, which was established in July 2001 and is funded by NICE to develop national clinical guidelines for nursing in the NHS. These types of guidelines and the standards that you adopt locally, either expressed in Trust-wide protocols or unit-based guidelines, become the quality standards against which I have suggested that you need to measure your performance. As a registered nurse, you will have a central role in developing and refining quality standards and appropriate measuring tools, along with multidisciplinary colleagues and patients themselves, through service user involvement mechanisms.

The emphasis on risk management is also relatively new to us in the UK and Alaszewski (2003) gives a clear account of how adverse events have shaped the NHS and led to such a loss of confidence that it was felt essential to adopt risk assessment and risk reduction programmes. We all know that accidents happen, but we must avoid the situation where we feel 'there is an accident waiting to happen'. You will be made familiar with risk assessment tools in your area and are probably familiar with some already ...

for dishonesty such as theft or fraud might well be deemed incompatible with the role and standing of a nurse. When I read these reports, I am often struck by the fact that there is rarely a single incident reported against a nurse; there is often a pattern of poor performance or conduct. So, if you feel that you or a colleague are 'struggling' to perform for whatever reason, remember that it is much easier to seek help and support as soon as a problem is spotted. Do remember that the vast majority of nurses will never come into contact with the NMC in such unfortunate circumstances and so we can usually concentrate on more positive aspects of the Council's work!

Summary

This chapter has included:

✔ **A look at the function of the NMC.**
✔ **Discussion of misconduct issues that reach the NMC.**
✔ **A detailed exploration of the competencies of the ONP.**
✔ **Reflections on possible differences between nursing practice in the UK and other health care systems.**
✔ **Some ideas for reading and activities to prepare you for nursing here.**

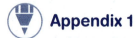 ## Appendix 1

NMC requirements for overseas nurses' programme leading to registration in the UK

Available at:
http://www.nmc-uk.org/aFrameDisplay.aspx?Document ID=917

Why don't you look these up? You can also look at the 'guiding principles' and content for the ONP.

1. Professional and ethical practice

● Manage oneself, one's practice, and that of others, in accordance with the NMC's code of professional conduct; standards for performance, conduct and ethics, recognising one's own abilities and limitations.

● Practise in accordance with an ethical and legal framework which ensures primacy of patient and client interest and respects confidentiality.

- Practise in a fair and anti-discriminatory way, acknowledging the differences in beliefs and cultural practices of individuals or groups.
- Demonstrate openness and acknowledge differences in between own culture and that in a multicultural UK.
- Demonstrate knowledge of the ways in which health and social care is established and delivered in the UK.
- Engage in, develop and disengage from therapeutic relationships through the use of appropriate communication and interpersonal skills.

2. Care delivery

- Understand and follow complex lines of argument in a health care topic.
- Read and understand new knowledge from articles in nursing journals.
- Effectively interact with a degree of fluency and spontaneity that makes information sharing with patients/clients and their relatives and colleagues possible.
- Actively participate in discussions about health care and patient issues, accounting for and sustaining personal views.
- Effectively report in writing and verbally, passing on information or producing reasoned justifications for actions in different situations.
- Engage in, develop and disengage from therapeutic relationships through the use of appropriate communication and interpersonal skills.
- Undertake and document a comprehensive, systematic and accurate nursing assessment of the physical, psychological, social and spiritual needs of the patients, clients and communities.
- Formulate and document a plan of nursing care, where possible in partnership with patients, clients, their carers and family and friends, within a framework of informed consent.
- Demonstrate sound clinical judgements across a range of differing professional and care delivery contexts.
- Based on the best available evidence, apply knowledge and an appropriate repertoire of skills indicative of safe nursing practice.
- Evaluate and document the outcomes of nursing and other interventions.

3. Care management

- Contribute to public protection by creating and maintaining a safe environment of care through the use of quality assurance and risk management strategies.

- Accurately interpret numerical data and their significance for the safe delivery of care.

- Accurately calculate and administer prescribed medication.

4. Personal and professional development

- Contribute to public protection by creating and maintaining a safe environment of care through the use of quality assurance and risk management strategies.

References

Alaszewski A (2003). Risk, clinical governance and best value: restoring confidence in health and social care. In: Pickering S and Thompson J (eds) *Clinical Governance and Best Value: Meeting the Modernisation Agenda*, Chapter 10. Edinburgh: Churchill Livingstone.

Allan H and Larsen J (2003). *'We Need Respect': Experiences of Internationally Recruited Nurses in the UK*. London: Royal College of Nursing.

Caulfield H (2002). Law: issues for nurses. In: Daley J, Speedy S, Jackson D and Darbyshire P (eds) *Contexts of Nursing*, Chapter 10. Oxford: Blackwell.

Chambers N (2002). Wound management. In: Hogston R and Simpson P (eds) *Foundations of Nursing*, Chapter 8. Basingstoke: Palgrave.

Clayton J (2003). Clinical governance and best value: a toolkit for quality, Chapter 1. In: Pickering S and Thompson J, ibid.

Cronin P and Rawlings-Anderson K (2004). *Knowledge for Contemporary Nursing Practice*. Philadelphia: Mosby.

Crookes, P, Griffiths R and Brown A (2002). Becoming part of a multi-disciplinary health care team. In Daley J *et al.*, ibid.

Department of Education and Skills (2005). *Skills for Life: Effective Communication for International Nurses*. London: DfES.

Dimond B (2005). *Legal Aspects of Nursing*, 4th edn. Harlow: Pearson Education.

Fletcher L and Buka P (1999). *A Legal Framework for Caring*. Basingstoke: Macmillan.

Gerrish K and Griffith V (2004). Integration of overseas nurses: evaluation of an adaptation programme. *Journal of Advanced Nursing* **45(6)**: 579-587.

Hardill I and Macdonald S (2000). Skilled international migration: the experience of nurses in the UK. *Regional Studies* **34(7)**: 681-692.

Jasper M (2002). Challenges to professional practice. Chapter 14. In Hogston R and Simpson P, ibid.

McSherry R and Taylor S (2003). Developing best practice, Chapter 5. In: Pickering S and Thompson J, ibid.

Oxford English Dictionary (1994). Buckingham: OU Press.

Parker S and Clare J (2002). Becoming a critical thinker, Chapter 17. In: Daly J *et al*, ibid.

Seedhouse D (2000). *Practical Nursing Philosophy: the Universal Ethical Code*. West Sussex: Wiley.

Seedhouse D (2005). *Value Based Decision Making for Healthcare Professionals*. West Sussex: Wiley.

Spector R E (2004). *Cultural Diversity in Health and Illness*, 6th edn. New Jersey: Pearson Prentice Hall.

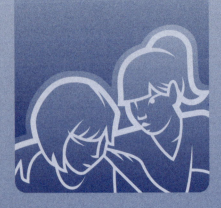

Chapter 3

How is health care in the UK funded and organised?

Ian Peate

This chapter will provide you with some essential background to the health care services of which you are going to be a vital part and enable you to:

- ✔ **Become aware of the structure and function of the National Health Service (NHS) and the Independent Care Sector (ICS) in the UK**
- ✔ **Consider the development of nursing as a profession**
- ✔ **Identify the nature and roles of various staff groups in UK health care**
- ✔ **Contrast the UK system with others with which you are familiar**
- ✔ **Consider the implications of those differences for your work here as a nurse**

There are approximately 60 million inhabitants in the UK and this is made up of citizens from various cultures and socioeconomic backgrounds (National Statistics Office 2005). The provision of health and social care for a country of this size, taking into account the multicultural makeup, is therefore going to be complex.

However, prior to gaining an understanding of health and social care delivery you must have an awareness and appreciation of both health care history in the UK and the proposed developments that will affect the care you deliver in a variety of settings with a range of patients. To develop an appreciation of contemporary British nursing practice, it is important to have an understanding of where nursing has come from, how nursing and the health service has emerged and how it continues to evolve (Craig and Daniels 2004). To contribute effectively to the delivery of health care you must have some understanding of the structure in which health and social care provision is organised, along with the people who are involved in the delivery of those services.

What is the NHS?

Prior to the setting up of the NHS in the 1940s, health care provision was a luxury available only to those who could afford it. Often those who could not afford health care—the poor, diseased and homeless—went without it. Hospitals charged for services and so charitable individuals and foundations had to work hard to ensure that those who needed care were able to receive it free of charge. Nursing grew out of domestic service in large houses and families, and many nurses in the original charitable institutions were rather like servants. Baly (1995) describes how they were often ignorant, unsuitable for the work and even drunkards! Most of you will be familiar with the work of Florence Nightingale, whose efforts led to the establishment of training programmes for nurses here in the UK, and then worldwide. However, we must remember that her first school was only opened in 1860, and so nursing is still relatively young compared to other professions.

People who were mentally ill or had a mental handicap (now called learning disability) were isolated in large asylums and institutions. This, it was said, was for their own good. In reality the conditions were often so bad that many patients became worse, not better. Elderly people were treated just as badly and often many died in institutions known as workhouses. There were no dedicated or preventative services for children, who were treated in ways that today would be regarded as cruel.

Health care provision was in need of reform. The NHS, which was established over 50 years ago, in 1948, is a large and complex organisation. The NHS is Europe's largest single employer and employs over 1.3 million people (Department of Health 2004).

Over the years the NHS has undergone numerous reforms and reorganisations in response to the ever changing health care needs of the population, advances in technology, and the management and care of people. The service continues to change and grow. The aim of the NHS is to provide health care for all citizens and the provision of health care today is based on need and not the ability to pay.

Three years after its creation the noble concept of a free-for-all service was challenged and the charging of modest fees for some services was introduced; for example, prescriptions and dental services. Charges for some services, for those who can afford them, still exist today. A popular phrase to describe the NHS was that it would care for people 'from cradle to grave', thus from the time of birth through all life's stages until death.

Activity

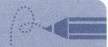

Consider the health care system known to you in another country. Is it free at the point of delivery? What do you think of free health care for all? Can you see any problems with such a system?

As the decades pass the NHS develops, grows and responds to the challenges it faces with an ever increasing need to improve cost consciousness. A white paper, a document produced by the Department of Health (DH) that lays down firm proposals for new law, proposed to improve the running of the NHS based on a partnership approach and driven by performance (Department of Health 1997) – *The New NHS: Modern and Dependable*. There are six principles associated with the new NHS:

- To renew the NHS as a genuinely national service, offering fair access to consistently high quality, prompt and accessible services right across the country.

- To make the delivery of health care against these new national standards a matter of local responsibility, with local doctors and nurses in the driving seat in shaping services.

- To get the NHS to work in partnership, breaking down organisational barriers and forging stronger links with local authorities.

- To drive efficiency through a more rigorous approach to performance, cutting bureaucracy to maximise every pound spent in the NHS for the care of patients.

- To shift the focus on to quality of care so that excellence would be guaranteed to all patients, with quality the driving force for decision-making at every level of the service.

- To rebuild public confidence in the NHS as a public service, accountable to the patients, open to the public and shaped by their view.

It has been over 50 years since the initiation of the NHS, and the aim is to place the patient at the centre of the service, with a shift in focus from a service that was predominantly a paternalistic system – doing things to and for patients – to one which works with patients.

How is care provided?

The NHS provides most health care in the UK, with other care providers (the independent sector – sometimes called the ICS or the private sector), also making a contribution to care provision. Predominantly these are UK-wide independent hospitals, clinics and nursing and residential homes. Just as the NHS is required to adhere to various Acts and Directives to provide support to patients and their treatment, so too is the independent sector; see, for example, the Health and Social (Community Health and Standards) Act 2003.

How is it funded?

The main source of funding for the NHS is general taxation paid by the residents of the UK. In effect the government becomes the single payer for health care, no additional costs are incurred through taxing from source, and it is an efficient method for raising revenue (Baggott 2004). As access to health care is not associated with the individual's financial contribution, the provision of care is based (usually) on the principles of clinical need – a concept that has been the basis of the NHS for over 50 years. However, one disadvantage of such a system is that it ties health services very closely to the state of the economy, as well as to the taxation policies of current government. Any changes in the economy, for example a recession, can threaten the health budget with ensuing consequences for services. Funds for health care, decided almost entirely by central government, must also compete with the requirements of other government-funded entities, for example, education, as well as additional demands made of government funds. However, the general taxation approach remains to this day; Wanless (2002) suggests it is the most efficient as well as the fairest system.

Private insurance is another method of health care funding; this can be used by individuals who may require a quicker or more responsive service. Currently, those with private health insurance are those who access private health care provision, which may provide a quick-to-respond service. However, there is no guarantee that this will be a better quality care service than that offered by the NHS. The underlying principle associated with private insurance (the independent sector) is that the ability to treat is closely related with the patient's ability to pay.

 # What is health and social care?

Means *et al.* (2003) state that most NHS expenditure is allocated to the care and treatment of:

- Elderly people
- Children
- People with mental illness

- People with learning disabilities
- Those with a chronic illness

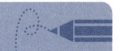

Activity

Are you surprised by this explanation of expenditure? Can you think of any reasons why it might be like this? Which care group receives most public funding in your country?

The essence of community care (where most of the provision of care for the above groups takes place) is that people should be looked after in their own homes and other non-institutional environments, as opposed to large institutions and hospitals (Payne 2000). In an attempt to enhance quality of life services provided to these groups of people by both, the health and social sectors are becoming more integrated. Joint working between social and health care professionals is vital if care provision is to be effective.

Generally, social services are run by local councils. For example, Liverpool City Council provides information, advice and social care to the people of the City of Liverpool. Each person in need of social services (supported living services) will have their needs assessed. Care packages, the result of in-depth assessment of need, may include help with personal care, i.e. help with hygiene needs, assistance with eating, and support with getting up and going to bed. The following services may be provided depending on assessment of need:

- Home (domiciliary care) and community support
- Day care services
- Intermediate care and rehabilitation services
- Supported housing
- Respite care
- Minor adaptations to the home
- Equipment loans

With regard to funding, care homes and residential homes are in a complex situation which is not always easily understood. Some such homes may be run and funded completely by local NHS funds, and some may be completely 'private' and residents may be paying for all their accommodation and care. The majority, however, will be a combination of the two and provide care for fee-paying and NHS clients. The issue of whether the NHS should pay for non-medical or 'social care' of elderly people is regularly debated by the public and politicians, and there are currently anomalies between the different member countries of the UK.

Various influential DH documents, for example, the National Service Frameworks (NSFs), have been produced to provide nurses and others with guidance and standards (see, for example, Department of Health 2001b – National Service Framework for Older People). The NSFs attempt to bring together and coordinate services that are provided by both the health and social care sectors.

What is the structure of the NHS?

The NHS plan, a document produced by the DH in 2000, detailed the biggest changes to occur in the NHS since its inception in 1948. A 10-year strategy was outlined in relation to reform of NHS provision. One other important feature that has occurred in the UK was the introduction of devolution; this is the process of devolving power from the centre to subnational units (Leeke *et al.* 2003). This has had an effect on how health care services operate in the four countries of the UK:

- Wales
- England
- Northern Ireland
- Scotland

Essentially, the NHS can be divided into two sections – one that deals with strategy, policy and management issues, and one that addresses all clinical aspects of care. The largest provider of health care in the UK is the NHS in England, and this section of the chapter will consider the structure of the NHS in England. The organisation of the NHS is unlike any other western health care system, and ultimate responsibility lies with the government and the minister with responsibility for health, the

Secretary of State for Health. It must be remembered, however, that each registered nurse, midwife and specialist community public health nurse is accountable for his/her own actions and omissions (NMC 2004). The system of organisation in the NHS is hierarchical in nature, with Parliament and the Department of Health at the top.

Parliament

Funds are allocated to the NHS in England through taxation and the Secretary of State for Health then decides how the funds are to be spent (Royal College of General Practitioners 2004). The Secretary of State is accountable to Parliament for the functioning of the NHS (Association of Clinical Pathologists 2005).

Department of Health

The DH is responsible for running and improving the NHS as well as pro-viding strategic leadership to both the NHS and social care organisations. Some of these responsibilities are outlined below:

- Setting overall direction
- Ensuring national standards are set
- Securing resources
- Making major investment decisions – investing in the service
- Improving choice for patients and users

(Adapted from: Royal College of General Practitioners 2004, Parker and Brooker 2004, Association of Clinical Pathologists 2005)

As well as the Secretary of State for Health there are five other Health Ministers who all work towards achieving the aims of the department. There are several other aspects associated with the DH; for example, the DH Board, Heads of Professions, National Clinical Directors and the Modernisation Board.

Official publications also make reference to 'arm's length bodies'. These are independent organisations that are sponsored by the DH to under-take its executive functions. Some of the arm's length bodies are directly related to, and have an impact on, the patient, the nurse and subsequent treatment; for example, the National Blood Service, National Patient Safety Agency, and National Institute for Health and Clinical Excellence (also known as NICE). These are Special Health Authorities.

Strategic Health Authorities

These authorities manage the NHS at a local level and feed back to the DH. The role of the Strategic Health Authorities (SHAs) is to support the efforts of the local health service by improving performance and integrating national priorities into local health delivery plans.

Where is this care delivered?

It is important to bear in mind that the majority of care provided to patients is carried out in the primary care setting. Take a look at Table 3.1 , which shows the settings for certain types of care. The three divisions are provided in what appears to be a distinct split; in reality the

Table 3.1 Examples of primary, secondary and tertiary care services

Aspects of care service provision	Examples
Primary care – those in the front line. Over 95% of care is delivered in the primary care sector by various health care professionals	• Dentists • General practitioners (GPs) • Pharmacists • Optometrists • Teams of nurses, midwives and specialist community public health nurses • Child psychologists
Secondary care – occurs mainly through the acute hospital setting. The nurses and medical staff providing care in this sector have more readily available access to specialist and elaborate diagnostic aids	Acute hospital settings with facilities such as: • X-ray departments • Operating theatres • Special care baby units • Microbiological/histological laboratory facilities
Tertiary care – this provision may be situated in large hospitals, providing the patient with highly specialist health care professionals dealing with particularly difficult or rare conditions	• Neonatal intensive care units • High dependency units • Burns units • Oncology centres • Specialist cardiac and transplant centres

(Royal College of General Practitioners 2004)

divisions between the sectors are becoming less distinct. The current government aims to break down the barriers between the primary and secondary care sectors, with an overall plan to enhance local decision-making and provide more patient choice (Department of Health 2001a).

Activity

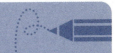

Are you surprised by this description of care settings? Where would you think most care is provided?

What are these different NHS Trusts?

Primary Care Trusts

Each Primary Care Trust (PCT) is responsible for the planning, securing and improving of primary and community health services in their local area. Their work is with patients, the public and GP practices. PCTs have the authority to commission health care services from secondary care providers and independent hospitals.

NHS Trusts

Most health service workers are employed by the NHS Trusts that run most of the hospitals in England. Their income is received via the commissions they receive from the PCTs. Included here are:

- Foundation Trusts – hospitals with special status, in essence, owned by members from the local community (Department of Health 2002).
- Mental Health Trusts – providing specialist mental health services in hospitals and the community.
- Care Trusts – designed to encourage the integration between health and social care sectors.
- Ambulance Trusts – providing patients with emergency access to health care, may also have the responsibility for providing transport for patients to and from hospitals for treatment.

What has been happening lately?

There are tangible moves towards making the NHS more responsive to the needs of the patient by providing the patient with alternative ways of accessing health services. It is important for you to have an awareness of them, not just because you might work there, but also because you need to understand the experiences of the patients you will be looking after.

NHS Direct

In March 1998 the government introduced NHS Direct, a convenient and alternative access to traditional GP services. This is a nurse-led health advice service providing the population with 24-hour health advice they can access over the telephone (08454647). This e-health approach has grown and expanded; it could be suggested that this is the world's largest provider of e-health services. The organisation manages and handles over half a million calls per month as well as providing approximately half a million online transactions via its web-based service on NHS Direct Online (**http://www.nhsdirect.nhs.uk/**).

NHS walk-in centres

Just as NHS Direct can be seen as an alternative method of accessing GP services, so too are NHS walk-in centres. In England these centres are increasing in number; they provide patients with fast and convenient treatment and advice in relation to a range of injuries and illnesses. They are staffed by experienced registered nurses. Minor illnesses such as colds, coughs and infections can be treated; minor injuries, for example, burns, cuts and sprains, can also be assessed and treated. Most of the centres are open from early in the morning to late at night, 7 days a week. One further advantage for the patient is that there is no need to make an appointment.

Who are the staff in the NHS?

This is one of the most important aspects of care provision for you to consider and learn about because the NHS has a wide range of staff groups in its employ, and you will be working or liaising with many of them! Table 3.2 provides a breakdown of the staff groups employed within the NHS, followed by an explanation of members of these groups.

Activity

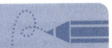

Before you look at the table, have a think about the groups and numbers of staff in your country. Are you surprised by the numbers of qualified health staff here? What do you think of all the speciality groups or roles? What implications do you think this diverse range has for health service management?

Table 3.2 Numbers of staff in the NHS and the groups to which they belong (Department of Health 2004)

Staff group	Number
Professionally qualified clinical staff	660 706
• Qualified nurses, midwives, health visitors (including practice nurses)	397 515
• Doctors	117 036
• Qualified scientific, therapeutic and technical staff	128 883
• Qualified ambulance staff	17 272
• Support to clinical staff	368 285
• Support to doctors and nursing staff 303 630	
• Scientific, therapeutic and technical support staff 55 025	
• Ambulance support staff 9 630	
• Staff involved in NHS infrastructure support	211 489
• GP practice staff (excluding practice nurses)	90 110

The strategic intentions of the current government for nurses, midwives and health visitors have been set out in the document *Making a Difference* (Department of Health 1999). The Royal College of Nursing (RCN) and the DH (Royal College of Nursing and Department of Health 2005) have produced their vision of the nurse working in advanced and extended roles.

Chief Nursing Officer

The Chief Nursing Officer (CNO) is responsible for ensuring that the government's strategies, for example, *Making a Difference* (Department of Health 1999), are achieved. This post holder is a civil servant and the most senior nursing and midwifery advisor. The CNO also has responsibility for some other AHPs.

Modern matron

The role of the modern matron is to support front line colleagues in the delivery of high quality care to patients. The matron provides leadership to staff associated with essential aspects of care, such as hygiene and dignity. The fundamental role is to improve the patient experience (Department of Health 2003). The matron's role was reintroduced in 2001 as a result of the NHS plan (DH, 2000). Modern matrons are located in both institutional and community care settings.

Nurse consultant

These nurses are senior nurses with much experience; they are expert practitioners. There are several nurse consultants in post who work within the hospital, also in the community, and across all nursing specialities: for example, Macmillan nursing (palliative care); gynaecology; endoscopy; infection control; child and adolescent mental health services (CAMHS); epilepsy; critical care; tissue viability.

There are four main areas of responsibility associated with the role of the nurse consultant (Department of Health 1999), with the overriding aim of strengthening professional leadership. They are:

- Expert practice
- Professional leadership and consultancy
- Education and development

- Practice and service development linked to research and consultancy

Most nurse consultants divide their time up into approximately 50% clinical practice, working with other nurses, health care professionals and patients, for example, managing and conducting their own clinics. The remaining 50% of their time is often spent undertaking research, teaching, leadership and evaluation activities (audit).

Ward sister/charge nurse/ward manager

Charge nurses are the male equivalent of the ward sister; collectively they may be known as ward manager. These senior nurses can be found working in all environments and across all nursing disciplines. As expert practitioners they have developed extensive skills and amassed a significant amount of clinical knowledge associated with their chosen area of practice. There are several features associated with the role of sister/charge nurse. The key aspects of the role are: to act as a role model, facilitate the learning of staff (nursing and non-nursing), manage a budget, assume overall accountability for patients nursed within their clinical area, and to be a competent and confident leader. Many of you may have held this or a similar position in your country of registration and may be interested to look for similarities and differences in the role.

Staff nurse

After successful completion of a minimum 3-year approved programme of study, the student nurse becomes a staff nurse. The approved programme of study is usually undertaken at a higher education institution. The staff nurse assumes full responsibility and is individually accountable for the care of a group of patients. This may be within a hospital or in the community setting. The nurse in the UK initially enters one spine of the Register only, for example, adult or children's nursing. To work as a registered nurse in another setting or speciality, further training is required. As the staff nurse consolidates his/her learning, becomes confident and gains more experience he/she may act as deputy for the ward sister/charge nurse. This is the professional grade and title to which you will be entitled once you have registered with the NMC. As is discussed in Chapter 7, there are a host of opportunities available after this initial registration.

Student nurse

All those who wish to become registered with the NMC must undertake and complete an approved programme of study. All candidates who wish to commence nurse education must satisfy the entry criteria set by the individual higher education institution. Currently, with respect to pre-registration nursing, there are two pathways the candidate may opt to undertake – the diploma and degree pathways. Both pathways lead to professional registration, but clearly have different academic qualifications attached.

All pre-registration nursing programmes provide the student with 50% of their time in practice (time spent in the clinical areas, both hospital and community) and 50% of their time undertaking theoretical work, usually based at the higher education institution (the university). The 3-year programme of study must be approved by the regulator, the NMC.

Activity

What do you think might be the advantages of having a choice of routes of study? How are nurses trained in your home country? Is nursing a popular choice there?

Medical staff

Consultant

Medical consultants can be found in a variety of settings, and the consultant has overall responsibility for the care of the patient. These doctors have undertaken further study, and are experts in their sphere of practice.

General practitioner

A member of the primary health care team, the general practitioner (GP) provides family health services to a local area in the community. The GP either works alone (a single-handed practice) or with other GPs (a group practice). GPs often treat patients themselves; however, there may be occasions when they refer patients to other doctors or nurses (i.e. consultants) or other health care professionals (e.g. physiotherapists).

Specialist registrar

The requirements of a specialist registrar are that they have completed a defined college or faculty specialist education programme. Once this programme of study is successfully completed, the doctor may be able to apply for a consultant's position if a post becomes vacant. However, if this is not the chosen route they may also take on more clinical responsibility and become a clinical assistant.

Senior house officer/house officer

When a medical student graduates from medical school as a house officer prior to registering as a doctor, he/she must undertake 1 year's hospital experience as a requirement of the General Medical Council (GMC). When registered with the GMC the doctor may apply to become a senior house officer. There are various clinical experiences available.

Medical student

The medical student in the UK will graduate (generally) with a Bachelor's degree in medicine and surgery (MB MS). Medical schools set their own entry requirements for those wishing to study medicine.

You are expected and, indeed, required to work as a member of the multidisciplinary team (NMC 2004). You will meet many other health care professionals and will be expected to work with them in a collaborative manner. This section of the chapter has focused on two groups of health care professionals only. Being aware of and understanding the roles and functions of other health care professionals can help you fully integrate and participate in effective health care provision for the patients you meet and care for. There has been great emphasis on the development of an integrated health care team approach, with all health care professionals aiming to provide patients with high quality care (DH 2000).

The NHS today is committed to the founding principles from over 50 years ago. The NHS:

- Meets the needs of everyone
- Is free at the point of delivery
- Is based on a patient's clinical need and not their ability to pay

Summary

In summary, this chapter has provided you with information that will enable you to:

✔ Outline a brief history of nursing and the NHS.
✔ Identify the management, policy-making and funding structure of the NHS.
✔ Discuss how care is provided outside the NHS.
✔ Discuss the different staff groups in UK health care.
✔ Reflect on how you will contribute within this huge enterprise!

References

Association of Clinical Pathologists (2005). *The ACP Guide to the Structure of the NHS in the United Kingdom*. East Sussex: ACP.

Baggott R (2004). *Health and Health Care in Britain*, 3rd edn. Basingstoke: Palgrave.

Baly M (1995). *Nursing and Social Change*. London; New York: Routledge.

Craig C and Daniels R (2004). Evolution of nursing practice. In Daniels R (ed.) *Nursing Fundamentals: Caring and Clinical Decision Making*, Chapter 1. New York: Thompson, pp. 2-23.

Department of Health (1997). *The New NHS: Modern and Dependable*. London: The Stationery Office.

Department of Health (1999). *Making a Difference: Strengthening the Nursing, Midwifery and Health Visiting Contribution to Health and Health Care*. London: DH.

Department of Health (2000). *The NHS Plan a Plan for Investment: A Plan for Reform*. London: DH.

Department of Health (2001a). *Shifting the Balance of Power Within the New NHS: Securing Delivery*. London: DH.

Department of Health (2001b). *National Service Framework for Older People*. London: DH.

Department of Health (2002). *A Guide to NHS Foundation Trusts*. London: DH.

Department of Health (2003). *Modern Matrons: Improving the Patient's Experience*. London: DH.

Department of Health (2004). *Staff in the NHS 2004*. London: DH.

Leeke M, Sear C and Gay O (2003). *An Introduction to Devolution in the UK*. Research Paper 03/84. House of Commons Library, London.

Means R, Richards S and Smith R (2003). *Community Care: Policy and Practice*, 3rd edn. Basingstoke: Palgrave.

National Statistics Office (2005). **http://www.statistics.gov.uk/** Accessed December 2005.

Nursing and Midwifery Council (2004). *The NMC Code of Professional Conduct: Standards for Conduct, Performance and Ethics*. London: NMC.

Parker J and Brooker C (2004). *Everyday English for International Nurses: A Guide to Working in the UK*. Edinburgh: Churchill Livingstone.

Payne M (2000). *Teamwork in Multiprofessional Care*. Basingstoke: Palgrave.

Royal College of General Practitioners (2004). *The Structure of the NHS: Information Sheet Number 8*. London: RCGP.

Royal College of Nursing and Department of Health (2005). *Maxi Nurses*. London: RCN.

Wanless D (2002). *Securing our Future Health Taking a Long Term View*. HM Treasury. London: The Stationery Office.

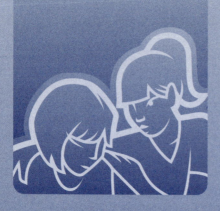

Chapter 4

What can I expect from my placement?

Philomena Shaughnessy

This chapter will look at placement and mentorship issues and will enable you to:

✔ Think about how you will achieve the learning outcomes in your placement
✔ Become aware of the educational audit system that covers placements
✔ Consider the role of the mentor
✔ Identify how you will solve any problems in your placement
✔ Explore your own role and responsibilities as a 'learner'

The NMC has determined that any ONP leading to registration in the UK must consist of two integrated parts, namely 20 days' protected learning time and a period of supervised practice, the length of which will be determined on an individual basis by the NMC (NMC 2005). This period is usually between 3 and 9 months, but will be calculated for you on an individual basis and notified to you by the NMC. We would strongly recommend that you do not leave your job or country of origin until you have received this NMC 'decision letter' and have obtained a placement.

Where will I be undertaking my 20 days' protected learning?

Your 20 days' protected learning time can be taken in either an educational setting, or in your supervised practice area. These are not to be seen as 20 'study days' but are intended to help you understand fully the content of the programme, explore your learning needs, and work towards the achievement of the required competencies. Some of these days may take the form of induction to practice in your supervised practice area and others might be structured days, taught in a university. Whatever the format of your protected learning, the most important thing to remember is that it should be meeting **your learning needs** i.e. the things that you need in order to achieve the competencies of the ONP. This means that you will need to take some degree of responsibility for your learning. You should identify your needs and then work out the objectives that will need to be fulfilled to ensure that these needs are met. Many nurses who are new to education in the UK find this a very difficult thing to do, as the extract below shows. However, it is a fundamental principle of adult education that learning needs are identified by the learner themselves. Don't forget that your mentor and your tutor at the HEI (higher education institution or university) will help you with this. Also, you are regarded as **supernumerary** (not part of the staff on duty for that day) during the period of protected learning, although not throughout the whole period of supervised practice. This supernumerary period is to enable you to be free to think about your learning needs and work out ways of fulfilling them without having to worry about completing various programmes of work.

Many of the trained staff, including your mentor, will advise you to take advantage of this time as, once you are qualified, there will be an expectation that you will be competent in the areas required by the programme. Even though there will always be training opportunities available, opportunities to explore your learning needs like this will be rare.

This is what one former ONP nurse said about placement learning:

I have found it quite difficult to have to take such a lead in my own learning. I thought that I would be told what to do, but my mentor expects that I will sit down with him and discuss my goals and learning needs. He has told me to take advantage of this time and ask for visits to other departments and to speak to nurse specialists and so on, because he says that when I am on the rota as a staff nurse, I won't get this opportunity.

 ## How can I be sure that I am going to a good supervised practice placement?

Your practice placement is arguably the most important part of your ONP; it is in practice that you will be able to gain the experience which will allow you to demonstrate your competence for registration in the UK.

Your supervised practice placement, the partner HEI, and the NMC must ensure that the kind of experiences that you need to fulfil these competencies are available to you, which means that all three will participate in a system of quality assurance.

This is achieved through a partnership between the HEI representative and the practice placement staff, and is measured by an **educational audit** of the placement each year.

All placements used for ONPs should also be suitable for providing practice experience to pre-registration nurses, so the same rigorous quality assurance processes in place for pre-registration nursing programmes will also be applied to placements used for the ONP.

What does this mean for me?

Essentially it means that the placement in which you will be under-taking supervised practice has been assessed as being of good quality and is able to give you a variety of learning opportunities which you can use to achieve your learning objectives, which in turn will enable you to achieve the competencies of the ONP.

All practice placements that are used as ONP placements are audited for quality annually by their partner educational providers. This involves several visits to the practice site by a representative of the HEI (often known as a link lecturer, or link tutor), who will work with the staff to ensure that learning opportunities are available in the placement which allow the competencies outlined in the ONP to be met.

The link tutor will use an audit tool which has been approved by the HEI to verify the quality of the practice placement. A copy of the audit will be kept in the placement and all staff and students can have access to it. Audit tools will vary in their layout according to the HEI; however, all are based on a set of guidelines laid down by the Quality Assurance Agency (QAA 2001). The audit will specify the following information as this is the minimum that the NMC requires:

1. An overall description of the environment.
2. The nature of the care that is being provided.
3. The number of patients being cared for.
4. The number of permanent staff in the placement and their designation and qualifications.
5. The experience of the NMC registered staff.
6. Identification of qualified mentors.
7. Information about the learning opportunities available in the placement, which is available to all staff and students.
8. The capacity for overseas nursing placements, which may include details of other students being supported by the placement.

Other important information about the placement

The Department of Health and the English National Board have published comprehensive guidance for education in practice for health care professions (Department of Health and English National Board 2001). This document provides a framework for assessing the quality of partnership between the HEI and placement providers and of the placement itself. Based on this guidance and, in addition to the information above, individual HEIs will normally seek out evidence of the following areas of practice.

- That the philosophy of care of the practice area is patient-centred, anti-discriminatory and empowering.
- That care provision respects the rights, privacy and dignity and cultural and religious beliefs and practices of patients.
- That high quality, evidence-based care is practised by all staff.
- That patients/clients are involved in the care process.
- Innovations in practice or care are developed and encouraged.
- That opportunities for multiprofessional learning are encouraged and developed.
- That clinical governance is practised as part of the quality assurance mechanism in the practice area.
- That there is a system of student evaluation and that the results of this are acted upon.
- The presence of learning material such as literature, internet access or other sources of contemporary information.
- That the continuing development needs of staff in the area are met. This may take the form of structured staff induction/training programmes to which other staff and students have access.
- That there is a high quality infrastructure which protects the health and safety of staff and patients.
- That mentors are adequately prepared for and supported in their roles, both as mentors and in the ONP programme.

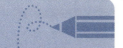

Activity

Ask if you can take a look at the audit for your placement area and see how all these points were measured and recorded.

In addition to educational audit, universities themselves are bound by the requirements of the Code of Practice of the Quality Assurance Agency for Higher Education. This Code of Practice covers all educational provision of universities, but has a specific section which covers practice learning (Section 9) (QAA 2001). This code requires that universities ensure the following.

- That placements are regularly quality assured by the HEI.
- The learning outcomes of placement learning are clearly defined and appropriate to the student's programme of learning.
- That practice assessment strategy is clear and coherent.
- That any professional body requirements are met, in this case NMC requirements for the ONP.
- That placement providers are aware of their responsibilities for the provision of learning opportunities, their role in the assessment of students and the health and safety of students.
- That students are aware of their rights and responsibilities in terms of managing their learning, their professional relationships and those towards patients/clients and other staff.
- That students are supported appropriately during the period of their placement learning.
- That there are systems in place to evaluate and act on the results of evaluation of placement learning opportunities.
- That there are policies in place to deal with complaints regarding practice placement.

As you can see, educational audit is a complex process which takes all facets of the learning environment into consideration when determining whether a placement is an appropriate place for any learner nurse to be gaining experience, upon which he/she will be basing his/her practice for a long time to come.

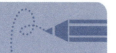

Activity

Look back both at the competencies that you are expected to achieve and at the educational audit for your placement. Can you see that you will be able to achieve these in your placement?

 ## What are my rights and responsibilities in my placement?

It is very difficult at first because you think that you don't know anything, but then you have to remember that you are a trained nurse and that you have so much valuable experience to offer. Some things are very different, especially the equipment, but my code of conduct is not so different from the code of conduct in use here, and patients are always glad of a helpful nurse. It is a strange situation because I am not a student nurse but I am not allowed to do the things that a staff nurse will do, and so it can be quite hard to know what I should be doing and this can cause me to worry.

Always remember that although in your country of origin you were fully accountable for your practice, you are not a registered practitioner in the UK until you have successfully completed your ONP and been entered onto the NMC register. Your responsibilities revolve around ensuring that you only undertake care that you are confident that you have the ability to do; identifying your learning needs appropriately and taking action to fulfil these needs. Conversely, if you feel that you are not progressing towards achieving your competencies, you must bring this to the attention of your mentor as quickly as possible and, with his/her assistance, make a plan to ensure that you are addressing the problems that you have both identified (see below). Remember, you must ensure that the care that you deliver abides by the principles laid out in the NMC Code of Conduct even though you are not yet registered.

As an ONP student you also have certain rights; these centre around the right to be supported by the HEI and your mentor. The things that you can expect from your mentor are outlined below. You also have the right to be treated in the same way as any other member of staff regarding your day-to-day working practices. In addition, there will be certain policies in place in your practice area that will be invoked in the event of a health and safety issue or in the event of a complaint against you or brought by you regarding the practice area, and you have the right to be protected by these in the same way as any other member of staff.

Activity

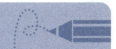

Think back to your experiences as a mentor or supervisor in your own country ... what makes for a good relationship between mentor and student? What have you expected from your students?

What can I expect from my mentor?

You may have gathered by now that your mentor is vitally important to you. He/she is the person with whom you will discuss your learning needs and who will help you resolve any issues or problems that you may encounter. He/she will also be the person who will conduct your interviews and assess you at the end of your programme.

Although all mentors are prepared for their role, they are also individuals and have slightly different ways of doing things, so don't be surprised if your experience is different from that of your colleagues. Provided you are achieving your learning objectives and discussing these and your competencies with your mentor regularly, all will be well.

Here are two differing experiences of being mentored:

When I started in my placement, my mentor told me that she wanted me to 'start as I mean to go on'. I didn't understand what she meant at first, but we talked about it and she was telling me to remember that I have got experiences as a nurse in managing a ward and so on, and that I should remember that in a few months I will be in charge here. So she expected me to take responsibility and learn from her role and watch how she manages the care assistants and other team members.

Although you have to do assessments and study to register as a nurse here, it is really important to remember that most of what you learn will come from working with trained staff and your mentor in your placement ... you really have to be able to concentrate and take in everything that you see every day, and keep asking questions if you don't understand why people do things differently, otherwise you might not get the chance again. Everybody is so busy, you have to make an effort to learn from them, and not always expect them to come to you with new things.

You will be allocated to an appropriately qualified mentor throughout the period of your supervised practice, and you must work with this mentor for at least 50% of your supervised practice time (2 days per week). An appropriately qualified mentor is a registered nurse who has had 2 years' experience post-qualification and has experience in the area of care relevant to your placement. The NMC are clear about what they expect of a mentor in terms of their duties towards any learner nurses who are assigned to them (Appendix 1). These are the result of a recent review of support for learners and introduce the role of 'sign off' mentor who will be ultimately responsible for confirming the fitness for practice of any learner who is about to enter the Register. Your mentor may also be a 'sign-off' mentor, or she/he may work closely with someone who is.

Activity

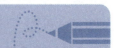

Read through Appendix 1 and think about your mentor. How does he/she fulfil these outcomes? How does this compare to the standards for mentorship in your home country?

Think about these domains and outcomes carefully, as many of these are as much about professionalism as a registered nurse as they are about mentorship. In any case, the Professional Code of Conduct specifies a teaching role for all registered nurses, so it is highly likely that you will need to fulfil these requirements in your own right, as a mentor to future students.

 ## What support does my mentor have?

All mentors have support from the partner HEI. Mentors are required to attend regular updates run by the HEI and they will also have support from the programme tutor and link lecturer (NMC 2002). Mentors should also have the support of the placement manager and/or care home owner, and should not feel that they are alone in trying to guide you.

 ## My mentor is too busy to work with me. What do I do?

Mentors are often extremely busy members of staff who are committed to teaching students, but also have other commitments to the practice area. It can be difficult for students to find a time when they feel that their mentor has enough time for them. Try to be understanding about this, whilst making sure that you get the time that you need and to which you are entitled. The NMC specify that you must work with your mentor for 50% of the time in a supervised practice placement. Although this equates to 2 days per week you can negotiate some flexibility in the arrangement with your mentor and placement manager. You may choose to work 4 days every 2 weeks, for example. This arrangement should work as long as there is another member of staff available to provide support in the interim. You will need to plan any holidays with the placement manager and mentor at the start of the placement so that you can work together. If you have any periods of sickness, this may extend your placement time.

This student explains how it feels to be a learner and talks about a way that she found of addressing this problem:

Sometimes I felt that the other staff just thought that I was a nuisance who was always asking questions. You do soon get used to it, though, especially if you really try to think about what you want to do beforehand and then talk it through with your mentor. After just a few weeks the staff did get used to me and I started to feel more confident; I was able to get on better with them. It is very difficult for nurses here who seem to have to spend a lot of time training and supporting nurses and students who are doing certificates and training. Looking back I can understand that they must have thought that I was just one extra person to look after!

In the same way as in your country of origin, professional behaviour includes being able to solve problems in a constructive way. If you are having difficulties, whether these are about lack of time spent with your mentor, or about any other practice-related issue, the first person to speak to about this is your allocated mentor. If she feels unable to resolve the issue, you must then speak to the placement manager, and also your link tutor so that the situation can be resolved as quickly as possible.

 I am going to be working with my mentor for 50% of my time in supervised practice. What happens if I need support at another time?

There will be other qualified staff working in your placement who will be able to support you. In some placements these are known as co-mentors, or supervisors. You should ask your placement manager who will provide you with additional support if you should require it.

 How will I know if I am making progress towards achieving my competencies?

Your mentor will hold an initial meeting with you to plan your supervised practice and discuss what you need to learn. You should expect this to be held shortly after the beginning of your period of supervised practice. At this initial meeting you should ensure that you go through the programme documentation together and that you understand how and when assessments will take place. Your mentor will hold at least three meetings with you in order to discuss and document your progress, and these are usually held at the beginning, midpoint and end of your placement.

The documentation from these meetings and the placement overall will vary according to your partner HEI, but it will include a record of your initial, midpoint and final meetings with your mentor; details of your protected learning time; the skills which you have learned or enhanced in your placement; and confirmation that you are competent to practice in the UK, which will be signed by your mentor or your 'sign off' mentor. This documentation will also need to be verified by the HEI who will then notify the NMC that you are competent to be entered on the Register. Therefore it is vital that you understand all of the documentation, that you have discussed it with your mentor, and that you ensure that it is completed accurately.

Do remember that even though your mentor may be very experienced, he/she will not know you very well and may not know too much about your skills and experience, so you must spend time thinking about this before the introductory meeting and then discussing this with him/her. You will then be able to plan your learning from the outset, and be clear about what is expected of you.

 ## What do I do if I think I am going to fail to achieve my competencies?

If at any point you think that you are not going to achieve your competencies, you must meet with your mentor as soon as possible so that you can make provision to gain the experience and guidance that you need. You may also need some support from the link tutor if this happens. You and your mentor should make a joint action plan with objectives to be achieved by you, which are related to the areas of practice which you are finding problematical. The action plan should also specify time scales that these objectives are to be accomplished in, and regular review dates. **Remember that you may only ask for one**

extension to your period of supervised practice from the NMC, so it is vitally important to ensure that you tackle problems in a positive way, and as soon as they are identified.

 ## What support can I expect from the partner HEI?

The partner HEI is there to support you and the practice staff in ensuring that you are helped to achieve the outcomes. You should expect to be given details of who to contact at the HEI and/or who will be coming to visit as link lecturer. Remember that the HEI is responsible to the NMC for assuring the quality of your experience. Thus, if you have any questions or anxieties that are not being addressed by your employer/placement provider, you must approach the HEI and be assured that the nurse teachers there will support you in seeking a solution. As an overseas nurse who is new to a placement, you may find it hard to voice complaints or queries but you do need to do so in a constructive way if you are to achieve your goals.

 ## What about supervised practice in different settings?

I am doing my supervised practice in a medical ward in a big NHS general hospital and my friend is doing hers in a nursing home which is in the independent sector

All care settings in the UK, whether they are part of the NHS or independently run, are subject to some form of quality assurance measure. For this reason the standard of care that they provide to patients/clients is expected to be high, and will enforce the values and standards which make up the competencies of the ONP. For example, practising in a professional and ethical way will require the same skills, attitudes and values whatever the care setting.

Generally speaking, the main differences that you will see if you are placed in a busy hospital is that patients will be admitted and discharged relatively quickly, either to and from home or to and from other care settings. Sometimes the problems that they are admitted with can be acute, requiring a period of intensive treatment before they are fit for discharge. This can mean that the staff will need some degree of specialist knowledge in a given area, for example, respiratory care. The medication that you are required to administer may be very different from that required by patients in different settings, but the principles of safe administration will be the same.

If you are placed in an independently run nursing or care home, you will find that patients/clients stay there for much longer periods of time, sometimes until the end of their natural lives, so the atmosphere needs to be as akin to home life as is possible.

Activity

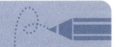

Are you accustomed to caring for patients in different settings, or have you only worked in hospitals? What sort of differences might you expect in terms of meeting your learning outcomes?

Both sets of patients will have similar needs for basic, yet high quality, nursing care, both sets of patients will be vulnerable, and will need a nurse with excellent knowledge and communication skills; it is simply the nature of how they are cared for that varies. It is easy to see that, although the tasks that you perform may be different, wherever this care is practised the basic principles will be the same. The NMC and the HEI and your mentor will need to be satisfied that you are competent in practising in an ethical, safe, professional and non-discriminatory manner, that you are able to assess, plan, implement and evaluate care for patients in whatever setting. This will require you to analyse information presented to you and reason with other professionals, and to communicate with patients and their relatives; therefore your communication, numeracy and analytical skills, both written and verbal, must be sufficiently well developed to allow this to happen. In addition, you will be required to understand risk, and implement and evaluate appropriate risk management strategies. Once again, the actual risks encountered in different settings will vary, but the principles required to deal with them will be the same.

Above all, don't forget that your mentor and other staff in your practice area are there to help you, and that even when you have passed the programme, all nurses need to keep themselves up to date in their own specialist area. Indeed, the NMC require that all nurses demonstrate that they have spent 15 days undertaking this every 3 years. Nobody knows everything about every setting; the idea is that you are able to demonstrate a set of principles that show that you are a competent nurse.

Summary

This chapter has provided you with an introduction to mentorship and placement issues, and you should be able to identify:

✔ **How your placement area will help you to achieve the learning outcomes through your placement experience and the 'protected learning time'.**

✔ **How the educational quality of placements is measured.**

✔ **What is expected of your mentor.**

✔ **How you and your mentor can work together to guarantee your experience meets your needs.**

✔ **Some tips for what to do if you feel you are not progressing.**

 Appendix 1

The following are extracts from the new *Standards to Support Learning and Assessment in Practice: NMC Standards for Mentors, Practice Teachers and Teachers*, which are effective from September 2007 (NMC 2006). Your placement will have a copy of the whole document for you to read, or you can obtain it online from the NMC website.

There is a single developmental framework to support learning and assessment in practice. It defines and describes the knowledge and skills registrants need to apply in practice when they support and assess students undertaking NMC approved programmes that lead to registration or a recordable qualification on the Register.

The NMC has identified outcomes for mentors, practice teachers and teachers so that there is clear accountability for making decisions that lead to entry to the Register. There are eight domains in the framework. The domains and related outcomes follow.

Establishing effective working relationships

- Develop effective working relationships based on mutual trust and respect.
- Demonstrate an understanding of factors that influence how students integrate into practice settings.
- Provide ongoing and constructive support to facilitate transition from one learning environment to another.

Facilitation of learning

- Use knowledge of the student's stage of learning to select appropriate learning opportunities to meet their individual needs.
- Facilitate selection of appropriate learning strategies to integrate learning from practice and academic experiences.
- Support students in critically reflecting upon their learning experiences to enhance future learning.
- Only mentors who have met the additional criteria to become a sign off mentor may assess proficiency.

Assessment and accountability

- Foster professional growth, personal development and accountability through support of students in practice.
- Demonstrate a breadth of understanding of assessment strategies and the ability to contribute to the total assessment process as part of the teaching team.
- Provide constructive feedback to students and assist them in identifying future learning needs and actions.
- Manage failing students so that they may either enhance their

performance and capabilities for safe and effective practice or be able to understand their failure and the implications of this for their future.

- Be accountable for confirming that students have met, or not met, the NMC competencies in practice. As a sign off mentor confirm that students have met, or not met, the NMC standards of proficiency in practice and are capable of safe and effective practice.

Evaluation of learning

- Contribute to evaluation of student learning and assessment experiences, proposing aspects for change as a result of such evaluation.
- Participate in self and peer evaluation to facilitate personal development, and contribute to the development of others.

Creating an environment for learning

- Support students to identify both learning needs and experiences that are appropriate to their level of learning.
- Use a range of learning experiences, involving patients, clients, carers and the professional team, to meet defined learning needs.
- Identify aspects of the learning environment which could be enhanced, negotiating with others to make appropriate changes.
- Act as a resource to facilitate personal and professional development of others.

Context of practice

- Contribute to the development of an environment in which effective practice is fostered, implemented, evaluated and disseminated.
- Set and maintain professional boundaries that are sufficiently flexible for providing interprofessional care.

- Initiate and respond to practice developments to ensure safe and effective care is achieved and an effective learning environment is maintained.

Evidence-based practice

- Identify and apply research and evidence-based practice to their area of practice.
- Contribute to strategies to increase or review the evidence base used to support practice.
- Support students in applying an evidence base to their own practice.

Leadership

- Plan a series of learning experiences that will meet students' defined learning needs.
- Be an advocate for students to support them accessing learning opportunities that meet their individual needs – involving a range of other professionals, patients, clients and carers.
- Prioritise work to accommodate support of students within their practice roles.
- Provide feedback about the effectiveness of learning and assessment in practice.

Mentors are responsible and accountable for:

- Organising and coordinating student learning activities in practice.
- Supervising students in learning situations and providing them with constructive feedback on their achievements.
- Setting and monitoring achievement of realistic learning objectives.
- Assessing total performance, including skills, attitudes and behaviours.
- Providing evidence as required by programme providers of student achievement or lack of achievement.
- Liaising with others (e.g. mentors, sign off mentors, practice facilitators, practice teachers, personal tutors, programme leaders)

to provide feedback, identify any concerns about the student's performance and agree action as appropriate.

- Providing evidence for, or acting as, sign off mentors with regard to making decisions about achievement of proficiency at the end of a programme.

References

Department of Health, English National Board for Nursing, Midwifery and Health Visiting (2001). *Placements in Focus. Guidance for Education in Practice for Health Care Professions.* London: ENB.

Nursing and Midwifery Council (2002). *Standards for the Preparation of Teachers of Nursing and Midwifery: Advisory Standards for Mentorship.* London: NMC. (Adopted from UKCC 2000.)

Nursing and Midwifery Council (2005). *Requirements for Overseas Nurses' Programme Leading to Registration in the UK. Circular 9 - Appendix 1*; 10th March 2005. London: NMC.

Nursing and Midwifery Council (2006). *Standards to Support Learning and Assessment in Practice: NMC Standards for Mentors, Practice Teachers and Teachers.* London: NMC.

QAA (2001). *Code of Practice for the Assurance of Academic Quality and Standards in Higher Education. Section 9: Placement Learning,* July 2001. Gloucester: Quality Assurance Agency for Higher Education.

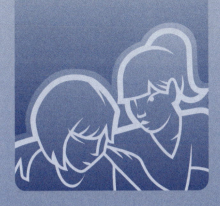

Chapter 5

What will it be like living and working in the UK? Introducing a multicultural workforce for a multicultural society

Jane Clapham and Kim Goode

This chapter aims to help you focus on issues of interest and potential concern as you prepare to start your career overseas. It will enable you to:

- ✔ Consider what is meant by the terms culture and multicultural
- ✔ Discuss why it is so vital for nurses to understand these issues
- ✔ Learn something of the culture and expectations of the people you will be nursing
- ✔ Take a look at yourself and your experience and decide what issues or difficulties you may have
- ✔ Decide on some preparations to lessen any difficulties or anxieties

Activity

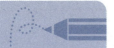

Firstly, read through and reflect on the following tale, and then contemplate the message.

The Greek Travellers

An old man was sitting by the side of the road one day, when a traveller came up and asked: 'What are the people like in the next town?'

'What were they like in the town you have just come from?' the old man asked in return.

'Awful', replied the traveller, 'rude and unfriendly'.

'Unfortunately' said the old man, 'I think you'll find they are much the same in the next town'.

A little while later, another traveller came up to the old man and asked the same question, 'What are the people like in the next town?'

'What were they like in the town you have just come from?' the old man asked in return.

'Great', replied the traveller, 'really polite and friendly'.

'Fortunately', said the old man, 'I think you'll find they are much the same in the next town' *(VSO 2003).*

What did you make of that? As nurses, we are lucky in that we are often welcomed wherever we work and are immediately part of a team in our work setting with the identity and comfort that may offer. However, it is important to think about how our attitudes and behaviour can affect the way in which we are received.

 ## Preparation for living and working in a different culture: what is it like in the UK?

You may have travelled here before, or you may already have friends or relatives working here, but how much do you really know about the UK

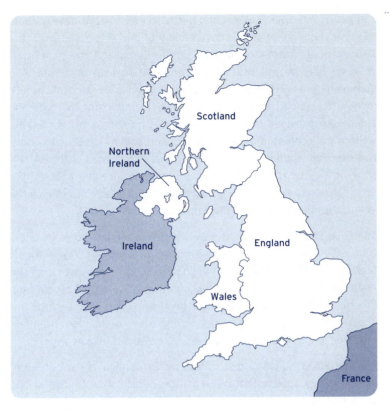

and its people? How much do you need to know? We have included a brief consideration of major population and religious groups in the UK, but remember that it is not exhaustive and is intended to encourage you to learn more.

Many people coming to the UK come from countries with a much larger land mass than this small set of islands. The UK is sometimes called Great Britain and is made up of four countries: England, Northern Ireland, Scotland and Wales. Although all their peoples will speak English as their first or second language, each country also has its own language and customs. The Republic of Ireland (the south of Ireland) is a distinctly separate country and there is a long and complex history regarding its relationship with England.

Each of our four countries has its own political assembly where laws which relate to this area are generated and administered. The three assemblies in Scotland, Wales and Northern Ireland have close connections with London, where the government for the UK is based within the Parliament of Westminster. Members of the European Parliament travel between the UK and Brussels (in Belgium) to help administer the European Union (EU). The UK has what is called a 'welfare state' where medical treatment, education and financial support for the poor and elderly are provided by the government. The money to pay for the welfare state comes primarily from the taxes paid by the British people. Not everyone within society receives equal experiences of the welfare state. It may be that disadvantaged groups include the people from ethnic minority groups. The government has strategies to reduce the inequalities in the provision of health care (Kingsley 2001).

The population of the UK has grown by 7% in the last 30 years or so, from 55.9 million in 1971 to 59.8 million in mid-2004 (UK National Statistics 2006, p. 32). Apart from English, Scottish, Northern Irish and Welsh people, the UK is home to an enormous diversity of people from other countries. Some of these have been here for several generations. These cultural groups are represented in every occupation, from law, medicine and politics to shopkeepers, carers and transport workers.

Helman (2000) suggests that culture can be defined as a set of guidelines within a society that governs how people view the world and behave towards one another, and which is passed between generations through art, literature and language. From this statement it can be seen that living within a society where a variety of people from different cultures coexist can sometimes be challenging. It also offers great opportunity for an interesting life which can lead to self-development.

 ## How can we 'define' culture and what it means to people?

Think about what might be cultural differences. This 'iceberg' exercise (cited in Lago and Barty 2003) helps you to identify those aspects of culture which are usually visible and those which are less visible.

Activity

Why don't you try the 'iceberg exercise' on yourself?

Make a note of aspects of life affected by culture ...

- List the things you might *see*
- List those that you cannot *see*

Amongst aspects that are noticeable, you might have listed things such as: people and their clothing, transport, food, houses, money, traffic, types of buildings, TV and media, advertising and leisure habits. We would expect you to identify things like educational qualifications, social class, social networks, relationships, divorce, non-traditional family networks, traditions, views on morality, religious beliefs, beliefs about health, illness, life and death, rituals and politics as amongst the less visible.

What are the key messages of this exercise? There are key messages both for you as a nurse and you as an individual. We would suggest that you think about the fact that cultures differ, yet there are similarities with your own. You will also have realised that this is called the iceberg because there is more hidden than visible and so, some cultural differences are easy to see whilst some have hidden aspects which need to be considered and may be an influence on those that you can see. Most importantly of all, when adapting to a new culture do not assume that you are aware of all these unseen influences.

Nursing within the UK really represents our multicultural society, with British nurses coming from every part of the world. A diverse group caring for a diverse group offers an opportunity for huge learning on both sides. Certain assumptions are made when nursing people of one's own culture, although this is not best practice. However, when looking after a group of patients from a variety of backgrounds and cultures, an open-minded, non-judgemental approach is essential. Respecting and trying to meet an individual's cultural needs is part of everyday nursing practice and is a clear part of the NMC Code of Professional Conduct (2002).

Activity

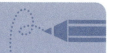

You might like to close your eyes for a few minutes and ask yourself:

'What are my cultural or ethnic prejudices?'

If a particular group come to mind, it would be valuable to explore the reasons for your feelings. Try to find out more about this group of people.

When preparing for your move abroad, it is important to prepare for the change of culture so that you are less likely to experience culture shock. Culture shock is a term for the psychological stress which travellers might experience because of differences between cultures and may be in response to the transition or change of cultures (the term was first used by Oberg 1960). It could be positive (as in surprise) or negative (as something occurs which is unexpected or disturbing). Homesickness and a desire to return home may also be a result of missing family and home or because of difficulty in adapting to the changes. Lago and Barty (2003) describe a whole cycle of contrasting feelings and experiences, and suggest that most people working or studying overseas will go through them. A common experience is to enjoy a 'honeymoon' period of enjoyment when you arrive, followed only weeks later by feelings of homesickness and isolation. Don't be surprised or disappointed with yourself if you find it harder to settle than you thought ... at the end of the chapter we will give you some more ideas about ways of preparing for and dealing with the changes.

 ## What is meant by diversity within the UK?

Types of family within the UK

One aspect of the diversity within the UK is the nature of how people choose to live together. The family is the basic unit of domestic living. There are several 'types' of family and some contain children and some

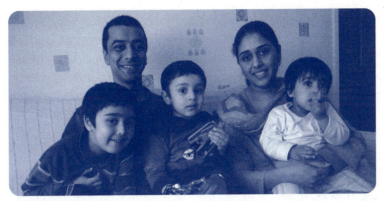

www.JohnBirdsall.co.uk

do not. A nuclear family consists of the father, mother and their children. This is the most common type of family, with over 80% of people living in this way in 2004 (UK National Statistics 2006, p. 1162).

However, other types of family are now quite usual. Many children are brought up by one parent. This may be the father or the mother and this family is called the single parent or lone parent family. Sometimes grandparents, uncles, aunts and cousins all live together with the parents and children. This would be called an extended family. A couple need not be a man and a woman; a couple can consist of two men or two women living together with or without their children. This is called a single gender family. In December 2005, the Civil Partnership Act (2004) came into being where single-sex couples can formalize their relationship with a ceremony which gives both individuals more rights, although it is not the same as a marriage (Office of Public Sector Information 2006).

Divorce and separation are not uncommon in the UK and people tend to form new families. This may mean that two parents may form a partnership and live together with their children from their former relationships. This can be couples of the same sex or a man with a woman. This family is often called a reconstituted family.

Some people also live in larger groups, perhaps in a very large house. This can be with or without children and is called communal living – sometimes in a commune or a community. In 2001, around a million people in the UK lived in this way (UK National Statistics 2006, p. 1162). Some of these are students living in residences, hotel or hospital employees living on the premises, boarding schools, residential homes or hostels for homeless people.

Many people also live alone in the UK. This is a growing trend with the ageing population. In 2004 there were 7 million people living alone in Great Britain, nearly four times as many as in 1961. The proportion of one-person households has more than trebled for working age people over the past four decades, while people of pension age were twice as likely to be living on their own. Three out of five women aged 75 years or over live alone (UK National Statistics 2006, p. 1162).

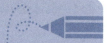

Activity

This is a very brief introduction to diverse family groups in the UK. Now consider your home country:

• Are there the same types of family structures?
• Do many people live alone?
• Even more importantly, why don't you take a few moments to think about the impact on nursing and care services of any of these structures that are new to you?

Are there many different cultural groups within the UK?

The 2001 Census revealed that the UK today is more culturally diverse than ever before (UK National Statistics 2006, p. 1311). The 4.6 million

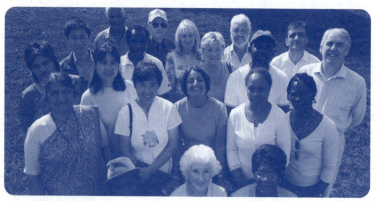

www.JohnBirdsall.co.uk

Table 5.1 Population of the UK by ethnic group, April 2001

	Total population (Numbers)	Total population (%)	Non-white population (%)
White	54 153 898	92.1	-
Mixed	677 117	1.2	14.6
Indian	1 053 411	1.8	22.7
Pakistani	747 285	1.3	16.1
Bangladeshi	283 063	0.5	6.1
Other Asian	247 664	0.4	5.3
All Asian or Asian British	2 331 423	4.0	50.3
Black Caribbean	565 876	1.0	12.2
Black African	485 277	0.8	10.5
Black other	97 585	0.2	2.1
All black or black British	1 148 738	2.0	24.8
Chinese	247 403	0.4	5.3
Other ethnic groups	230 615	0.4	5.0
All minority ethnic population	4 635 296	7.9	100.0
All population	58 789 194	100	

http://www.statistics.gov.uk/CCI/nugget.asp?ID=764

people from a variety of non-White backgrounds are not evenly distributed across the country, but tend to live in the large urban areas. The different groups share some characteristics but there are often greater differences between the individual ethnic groups than between the minority ethnic population as a whole and the white British people.

Although the expansion of the European Union in May 2004 initiated an increased inflow of non-British EU citizens to the UK, the majority of the UK population in 2001 were white (92.1%). The remaining 4.6 million (or 7.9%) people belonged to other ethnic groups (UK National Statistics 2006, p. 764; see Table 5.1).

Around half of the non-white population were Asians of Indian, Pakistani, Bangladeshi or other Asian origin. A further quarter were black, that is black Caribbean, black African or other black. Of the non-white population, 15% were from the mixed ethnic group. About a third of this group were from white and black Caribbean backgrounds. There were almost 691 000 white Irish people in the UK, accounting for 1% of the population (UK National Statistics 2006, p. 764).

In the UK the number of people who came from an ethnic group other than white grew by 53% between 1991 and 2001, from 3.0 million in 1991 to 4.6 million in 2001. In 1991, ethnic group data were not collected on the Northern Ireland Census (UK National Statistics 2006, p. 764). The non-white population of the UK is concentrated in large urban centres. Nearly half (45%) lived in the London region in 2001, where they comprised 29% of all residents (UK National Statistics 2006, p. 1306).

What about gender and age issues?

Amongst the people who come to live in the UK there is a diversity of behaviours between people; for example, men and women. Women in the UK generally see themselves as completely equal to men. Where it used to be that men 'looked after' women, many women would now regard themselves as independent. The 'liberation' of women has been developing since the World Wars of the 20th Century and has meant that many professions are now half (or more than half) women. An example of this is students entering medical schools. In 2002, 60.8% of those accepted into UK medical and dental schools were women (Royal College of Physicians 2004).

The pattern of the population in the UK is changing slowly. There are fewer young people and a higher number of older people. The proportion of those aged 65 years and over increased from 16% in 1971 to 19% in 2004. This figure is projected to rise to 23% in 2031 (UK National Statistics 2006, p. 1308). This means that many of our patients and

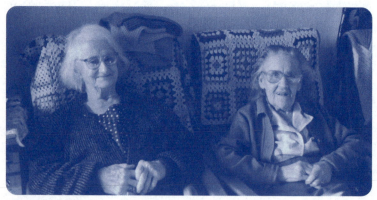

www.JohnBirdsall.co.uk

clients are elderly and this poses particular challenges for care services if their needs are to be met.

The proportion of people aged 85 years and over in the population has increased from 0.9% in 1971 to 1.9% in 2004 (UK National Statistics 2006, p. 1308). This will affect the population of those of working age. This working age group is shrinking, as those born during the 60s 'baby boom' move into retirement and are replaced by the adults from lower birth rate periods since the 1970s (UK National Statistics 2006, p. 1308).

The elderly in the UK do not mirror the cultural diversity of the younger groups, as some groups have been here longer than others (UK National Statistics 2006, p. 1263). A significant number of immigrants also move out of the country after staying here a while. Just over a third (34%) of foreign-born migrants who came to the UK in the 1990s emigrated within 4 years of arrival. Some elderly people in the UK are from the Caribbean, because of the large scale immigration to the UK in the 1950s. They have an older population on average than the UK-born Caribbean population (with ratios of 45.6 and 30.7 older people per 100 of working age, respectively, in 2001). The Republic of Ireland had as many as 65.9 older people per 100 of working age in the UK in 2001, reflecting immigration from the 1950s and earlier (UK National Statistics 2006, p. 1312).

The mortality statistics include details of the age at which people die. Differences in mortality rates mean that women aged 65 years and over normally outnumber men. In the white, mixed and Chinese ethnic groups the women outnumber men in the over 65 age group. However, for some ethnic groups this has been affected by differing immigration patterns. In the Bangladeshi population only a third of this age group are women. Similarly, women from Pakistan are outnumbered by men in this age group (UK National Statistics 2006, p. 456).

Religious diversity within the UK

We, as nurses, are concerned with providing culturally sensitive care for our patients and clients. However, it cannot be assumed that a Jewish patient, for example, needs a kosher diet or that a Muslim patient needs a Halal meal. Rather, we need to maintain an open mind and assess each person's needs as those of a unique individual. It is useful to understand the values and norms of the various religions practised within the UK, but stereotypical thinking should be avoided.

Activity

Consider the mix of peoples in your home country:

How many different religions are practised?

How are children educated with regard to their religion?

Is there any religious intolerance in your country?

What challenges does religious diversity present for nurses?

The religion question was the only voluntary question in the 2001 Census, and 8% of people chose not to state their religion (UK National Statistics 2006, p. 954).

Christianity

Christianity is the main religion in Great Britain. There were 41 million Christians in 2001, making up almost three-quarters of the population (72%). This group included the Church of England, Church of Scotland, Church in Wales, Catholic, and all other Christian denominations (UK National Statistics 2006, p. 954). These groups within the other Christian denominations are various and diverse. They include Methodists, Baptists, Seventh Day Adventists, Mormons (The Church of Jesus Christ of Latter Day Saints), Christian Scientists, Salvation

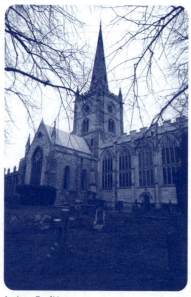

Andrew Fox/Alamy

Army, Jehovah's Witnesses, Quakers, Orthodox and Presbyterians. All of these groups hold to the belief that God was made manifest in a human being, Jesus Christ, over 2000 years ago.

People with no religion formed the second largest group in the 2001 Census, comprising 15% of the population. Often people coming to this country from overseas find this interesting, as it may be quite different in their own country (UK National Statistics 2006, p. 954).

Islam

About one in 20 (5%) people belonged to a non-Christian religious denomination. Muslims were the largest religious group after Christians. There were 1.6 million Muslims living in the UK in 2001. This group comprised 3% of the total population and over half (52%) of the non-Christian religious population (UK National Statistics 2006, p. 954).

The relationship between Christians and Muslims has a long and diffi-cult history. Both religions (and indeed Judaism) originally sprung from Abraham, living in Palestine before time was measured. One set of descendents became Jews, another became Christians and the third set became Muslims. Islam follows the teachings of God as given to Muhammad (peace be upon him) directly in the Koran. These teachings include God as a single entity. Islam is about surrender to God and God's will (Huston Smith 1991). An example of a difference between Christian women and Muslim women is that some Muslim women will wear some form of covering for their face. This is part of the Islamic practice of

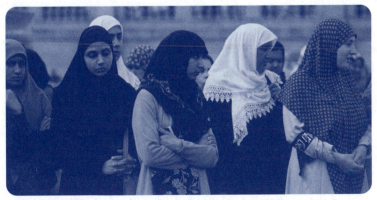

Geoff A. Howard/Alamy

purdah, the segregation of men and women. The covering is called a burqa and may or may not include a yashmak or veil to cover the face and sometimes even the eyes (Arif 2005).

Hinduism

Hindus were the second largest non-Christian religious group in the 2001 UK Census. There were over half a million Hindus (558 000), comprising 1% of the total population and 18% of the non-Christian religious population (UK National Statistics 2006, p. 954).

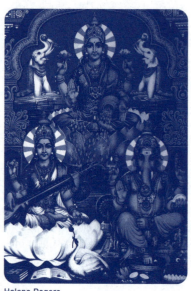

Helene Rogers

Hindus have a rich and luscious religion which involves the worship of more than one God. There are four Yogic paths which, if followed, all lead to union with the Divine. These are Bhakti Yoga, Jnana Yoga, Raja Yoga and Karma Yoga (Huston Smith 1991). Hindus are vegetarians and revere many animals, including the cow. Their personal standards involve washing in running water – bathing can be quite unpopular.

Sikhism

There were just over a third of a million Sikhs (336 000) in the 2001 Census, making up 0.6% of the total population and 11% of the non-Christian religious population (UK National Statistics 2006, p. 954).

Sikhism is an offshoot of Hinduism, but both religions (and also Islam) are noted for the importance of the family. The father is the head of the family and marriages are often arranged by the parents. Sikhism is similar to Hinduism in the importance of worshipping God and providing selfless service. The Sikhs believe in reincarnation and encourage mysticism. Sikhs believe in one God. They also believe in equality and pay no heed to the differences of creed or caste (Huston Smith 1991).

Baptised Sikhs are of a more spiritual order. They then enter the 'Khalsa' and carry upon their person a comb, a dagger, a particular undergarment and also a steel bangle. Their hair remains uncut for life. These five distinctions are called the five Ks and they remind the follower of his commitment to a holy life. The five Ks act as a constant reminder of their commitment to their particular spiritual path (Huston Smith 1991). These five symbols must not be removed, which makes it interesting when preparing a Sikh person for operating theatre.

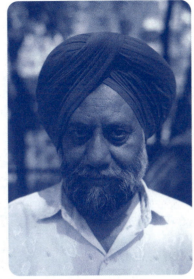

David R. Frazier Photolibrary, Inc./Alamy

Judaism

There were just over a quarter of a million Jewish people (267 000), constituting 0.5% of the total population and 9% of the non-Christian religious group (UK National Statistics 2006, p. 954).

It appears that the Jewish people were the first people to want there to be meaning in every event, who looked for the learning opportunity

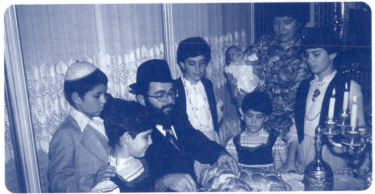

Rex Features

within each experience. It seems that this theology (as well as that of the Greek philosophers) has had a significant influence on western ideas of sociology and social policy. Ritual enables a person to identify themselves with a particular group, to feel as if they 'belong' to this group. Ringlets, caps, shawls and particular women's rituals in Judaism are some of the features that facilitate this. Ritual therefore can also enable members of a group to recognise each other (Huston Smith 1991).

Buddhism

Buddhists numbered 149 000 people in 2001, comprising 0.3% of the population of Great Britain (UK National Statistics 2006, p. 954).

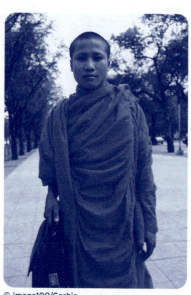

Siddhartha Gotama was born a prince in northern India around 500 BC. The Hindus believe this man was a reincarnation of one of the Hindu Gods, Vishnu. His life led to a spiritual path which resulted in his 'Great Awakening'. Buddha taught the philosophy of the four noble truths and the eightfold path as

© image100/Corbis

the means to awaken from suffering, and the virtues of compassion. Buddhism illustrates sharp insights into human behaviour, and teaches kindness and compassion. There are three slightly different groups of Buddhists: Theravada, Mahayana and Zen (Huston Smith 1991).

What are the implications of this diversity for nurses?

To avoid cultural generalisation, a useful approach may be to consider each situation and the patient and their individual needs. The following quotes and exercises will start to help you to consider some of the nursing differences when planning to nurse within a different working culture.

The difference in the organisation of health care work and nursing roles is highlighted by a Hungarian nurse who has recently come to work in the UK:

The UK is very friendly but is organised completely differently. In our hospitals in Hungary we do not have temporary or bank staff, only permanent staff. I am used to looking after so many more patients and we are given much bigger responsibility such as giving intravenous drugs and taking blood ... In the wards where I worked the patient usually stayed longer than 3 days so there was more contact. Szolnoki (cited in Bernard 2006)

An alternative perspective regarding coping with a different organisation of health care is illustrated by the comments from one mentor regarding overseas nurses:

They're generally not used to the fast pace of work, the turnover, the liaison with other professionals, other departments. It's hectic. You need to juggle these priorities the whole time. The overseas nurses find it hard to prioritise their work at first, because it's so different from what they are used to. (Gerrish and Griffith 2004)

An incident related by Widdrington (2006) illustrates a different point. A nursing student was 6 months' pregnant and working on a children's ward. This student nurse met the parents and grandparents of her young patient. All of the family shook hands with her, apart from the child's father. He put his hands behind his back and stepped away. Their relationship from that moment became 'difficult'. When the student mentioned this incident to a group of fellow students, one mentioned that in some cultures a man may not touch a pregnant woman who is not his wife. This insight helped the student to understand more about the family and she found ways of effectively communicating with the child's father about his son's care.

With regard to cultural awareness, a refugee from Somalia comments on her UK nursing experiences:

I currently work at [named] hospital and am interested in the way that multicultural care is delivered by different nurses to different patients. Patients are cared for respectfully, attention is paid to their cultural needs. For example, Muslim patients are offered Halal food; Jewish kosher and Hindu vegetarian. In my country we do not have this attitude and I am very impressed by the way that different cultures are recognised and respected here in London. Yaasen (2006)

 ## Understanding cultural needs and differences

As we have already stressed we do not wish to offer a 'handbook' for cultural issues, nor to suggest that there is any proper alternative to individual assessment, but it might be useful to look at some key areas, since appreciating the differences will be key to meeting needs.

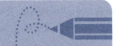

Activity

Consider each point below and examine the differences with your own culture or experience ... What are the implications for nursing care?

- Different ethnic groups may have different disease patterns. For example, people born in the Indian subcontinent have a high risk of coronary heart disease, whereas people of Afro-Caribbean origin have a high mortality rate from cerebrovascular accidents. Children born to Pakistani-born mothers have a higher risk of infant mortality (Naidoo and Wills 2001).

- Patients who have a strong religious belief may feel it should influence their decision-making on their care. For example, abortion is prohibited by Roman Catholics, organ transplantation is not permitted in the Buddhist faith, Jehovah's Witnesses forbid blood transfusion and organ donation (Spector 2004).

● Patients with strong religious beliefs may be sensitive to particular aspects of nursing or hospital care. For example, some orthodox Hindu women may not expose their bodies even when bathing (Naidoo and Wills 2001). Showering in running water may be preferable to baths for some Asian patients and Muslims. Gender issues may be of concern for some people, such that a female patient may refuse to be cared for by a male nurse, while others may find the open-backed theatre gown unacceptable (Mootoo 2005).

● Views of health may be seen differently by different ethnic groups; for example, traditional or herbal remedies may be taken rather than prescribed medications (Naidoo and Wills 2001). Different types of food are eaten for different diseases to restore health (Spector 2004).

● Beliefs about lifestyle issues may be very different; for example, alcohol and drugs may be forbidden for some people who follow the Baha'I faith. Some followers of the Hindu religion may not eat meat. Pork and alcohol are prohibited by the Islamic faith (Spector 2004). In Islam, people fast from sunrise to sunset during the month of Ramadan, although there may be different considerations if someone is sick.

● People from different cultures may have strong beliefs about pregnancy and birth rituals; for example, circumcision is performed on the 8th day for Jewish baby boys, and amulets may be placed on the baby in the Greek Orthodox faith. In China, fathers are not encouraged to attend the labour or birth of the baby (Spector 2004). Views on contraception may be strong, such as some Buddhists and Jews do not agree with contraception or family planning (Mootoo 2005).

● Patients from different cultures may have strong religious preferences about death, rituals and mourning. Some Islamic relatives will want the body washed by a Muslim of the same gender and, similar to the Jewish faith, the body must be buried as soon as possible. For people from Ireland there is a

practice of watching over the body to ward off any evil spirits
(Spector 2004).

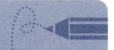

Activity

**Have you made a note of any differences? How would you find out
about religious needs and preferences of any group with which
you are unfamiliar?**

In addition to cultural differences amongst your future patients and
their families and friends, there are also cultural differences in the
organisation and philosophy of care which are equally important for
you to think about. Chapter 3 will give you an outline of the complex
organisation that is the NHS and it will be clear from this that both the
NHS and independent care sector are constantly changing and developing. Some of these changes are due to technology. Patients stay less
time in hospital, resulting in a high turnover of patients and everyday
use of advanced technology and different machines. Much of our
modern day equipment is disposable and equipment may be discarded
rather than reused.

Some of the reading on demographic patterns will have alerted you to
the fact that the UK has an ageing population, and many old people live
alone or in residential homes. This means, of course, that these people
may become patients with few visitors or social networks. What impact
does this have on care services? Some overseas nurses may be surprised at the lack of input from families in direct care-giving since,
except in the case of children, it is unusual for relatives here to wash
patients or provide food or bedding.

It is also true that many patients are very well informed about their condition after searching the web, and may require a much higher level of
information than you are accustomed to giving. Indeed, the government is very keen to ensure more patient (or service-user) involvement,
both in individual care decisions and in service organisation and management (Department of Health 2001). You may come to feel that
nurses and hospitals/homes are under scrutiny on issues such as hos-
pital-acquired infections owing, in part, to media involvement. This may

lead to patients or families asking you to justify or explain your actions in a way that you are not expecting. These are cultural differences in the philosophy and organisation of care and, as is obvious from the quotations by overseas nurses in this chapter, will be just as important for you to consider as issues around individual needs.

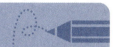

Activity

Can you start to see the challenges you might face in adapting to a different nursing culture? How can you prepare for these challenges?

Start to consider what you need to do to make this transference of cultures as easy as possible. Consider each point above and plan which one might be relevant to your clinical area and plan how you will find out more.

 ## How can you prepare before you come to the UK?

Consider your language skills; although your English language skills may be up to the acceptable standard (IELTS 7.0), you may need to consider that within the UK there are many different accents or dialects to understand, so listening to the radio and, in particular, the BBC world service may help your listening and comprehension skills. Reading British nursing journals will also help you to appreciate the jargon used every day in nursing. Reading a clinical skills book may also help, such as Dougherty and Lister (2004). Practise your English language skills as much as you are able. Overcoming language barriers was seen as vitally important for nurses from Korea settling into the US health care system; over time, non-verbal skills were also adopted (Yi and Jezewski 2000). You might also like to talk to people who have visited or worked in the UK and talk to any nurses who have studied or worked in the UK. You could also research the area/town/city in which you plan to live and find out about the population diversity in that area.

What about adjusting to a new living and studying/working culture?

Once you are here you could write a reflective journal/diary to understand the differences/challenges and what you could do differently next time. You might also build up networks to discuss issues with colleagues in your own language; the Royal College of Nursing (RCN) might be able to put you in touch with an Association of Nurses from your own country. *Do* prepare for times of homesickness/loneliness so plan a distraction, such as finding a market or shop which has similar food to your home, and keep contacts with home by email, letter and phone or by reading local papers, listening to local radio or TV via the web. If you practise a religion, then the local place of worship would be a useful place to meet new contacts as well as meeting your spiritual needs. Public libraries advertise local events, clubs and activities that might be of interest to you.

Do you remember the Traveller's Tale at the start of the chapter? We have a saying in English; that is, 'you will get as much out of this as you put in', which is a way of saying that, if you make positive efforts to adjust and adapt to your new life, then you will enjoy it much more!

 ## What can be learned from an overseas experience?

An overseas nurse working in the UK makes this observation:

In my home country, in Africa, people with dementia, they're not treated well. We don't understand their needs ... in the future I'd like to go back to my home country and develop better services for dementia patients. There's much to be done. **(Gerrish and Griffith 2004)**

Equally, do remember that you may be an expert nurse in your area of practice and, once settled, you may be able to develop and enhance nursing care here ... the learning goes both ways! The benefits and insight when working in a different culture may allow the sharing of ideas and experiences and develop understanding between groups of people, which can only benefit patient care.

Summary

This chapter has introduced you to some of the issues around multicultural Britain and has offered you the opportunity to:
- ✔ **Look at major demographic patterns in the UK.**
- ✔ **Consider some of the major religious and cultural groups here.**
- ✔ **Think about how you feel about nursing in this society.**
- ✔ **Think about how you will deal with the changes this entails.**
- ✔ **Prepare yourself for your adventure!**

Suggested further reading or contacts

Clinical nursing skills books such as:

Dougherty L and Lister S (2004). *The Royal Marsden Hospital Manual of Clinical Nursing Procedures*, 6th edn. Oxford: Blackwell.

Different cultures and religions booklet such as:

Mootoo JG (2005). A guide to spiritual awareness. *Nursing Standard* **19(17)**. [Now published by RCN Publishing Company.]

Nursing journals such as:
Nursing Times, found at:
http://www.nursingtimes.net/
Nursing Standard, found at:
http://www.nursing-standard.co.uk/
Professional Nurse, found at:
http://www.professionalnurse.net/nav?page=pronurse
Journal of Advanced Nursing, found at:
http://www.journalofadvancednursing.com/

Keep up to date with latest news:
Guardian newspaper, found at:
http://www.guardian.co.uk/
Times newspaper, found at:
http://www.timesonline.co.uk/uk/
BBC News service, found at:
http://news.bbc.co.uk/
BBC world service, found at:
http://www.timesonline.co.uk/uk/

Royal College of Nursing, found at:
http://www.rcn.org.uk/

References

Arif Z (2005). A question of gender. *Multicultural Nursing* **1(3)**: 12-13.

Bernard A (2006). Welcome to the club. *Multicultural Nursing* **1(4)**: 14-15.

Department of Health (2001). *Shifting the Balance of Power Within the New NHS: Securing Delivery*. London: Department of Health.

Dougherty L and Lister S (2004). *The Royal Marsden Hospital Manual of Clinical Nursing Procedures*, 6th edn. Oxford: Blackwell.

Gerrish K and Griffith V (2004). Integration of overseas nurses: evaluation of an adaptation programme. *Journal of Advanced Nursing* **45(6)**: 579-587.

Helman CG (2000). *Culture, Health and Illness*, 4th edn. Oxford: Butterworth Heinemann.

Huston Smith G (1991). *The World's Religions: Our Great Wisdom Traditions*. San Francisco: Harper.

Kingsley S (2001). Creating a climate for diversity and race equality in health care. *Ethnicity and Health* **6(3/4)**: 255-263.

Lago C and Barty A (2003). *Working with International Students: Cross-cultural Training Manual*. London: UKCOSA.

Mootoo JG (2005). A guide to spiritual awareness. *Nursing Standard* **19(17)**. [Now published by RCN Publishing Company.]

Naidoo J and Wills J (2001). *Health Studies: An Introduction*. Hampshire: Palgrave.

Nursing and Midwifery Council (2002). *Code of Professional Conduct*. London: NMC.

Oberg J (1960). Culture shock: adjustment to new cultural environments. *Practical Anthropology* **7**: 177–182.

Office of Public Sector Information (2006). http://www.opsi.gov.uk/ACTS/acts2004/20040033.htm

Royal College of Physicians (2004). http://www.rcplondon.ac.uk/college/statements/briefing_womenmed.asp

Spector RE (2004). *Cultural Diversity in Health and Illness*, 6th edn. New Jersey: Pearson Prentice Hall.

UK National Statistics (2006).

http://www.statistics.gov.uk/default.asp

Voluntary Services Overseas (VSO) (2003). *Preparing for Change Trainer Guide November*. London: VSO.

Widdrington C (2006). Improving your cultural awareness. *Nursing Times* **102(9)**: 40–41.

Yaasen L (2006). Aspiring to nurse. *Multicultural Nursing* **1(4)**: 39.

Yi M and Jezewski MA (2000). Korean nurses' adjustment to hospitals in the United States of America. *Journal of Advanced Nursing* **32(2)**: 721–729.

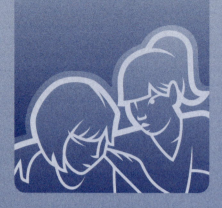

Chapter 6

Communication skills and 'UK health care English'

Theo Adris-Gilbert and Siegrid Beck

This chapter will look at the communication and language tasks that you will need to consider and explore the accompanying skills that you will require. You will be able to:

- ✔ Think about the importance of effective communication, especially for nurses
- ✔ Consider how language and other skills contribute to effective communication
- ✔ Identify key tasks that might provide challenges, such as patient admissions
- ✔ Identify priorities for your own language development
- ✔ Explore strategies to meet some of the language challenges

When you start working in the UK health care work place, you might feel overwhelmed by the many different tasks you are expected to do as well as the rules, forms and policies with which you must work. At the same time, you will have to deal with it all in 'UK health care English'. Understandably, you may feel that there is some pressure on you. You are right! But our first advice to you is *stop worrying*. Remember, if you are reading this, it is likely that you speak at least one other language and possibly more. Many of your patients and colleagues will only speak English. Your skills are therefore strong right now as a linguist. You are simply going to develop further the skills you are already lucky enough to have. For some of you, English will be a first language but, even so you will need to remember that effective communication is not just about the words you use, but about how you use them, tone of voice, body language and so on, and that may be different from your home country. Good luck!

Good communication skills are so very closely linked to your own personal and social skills that it is sometimes difficult to measure which of these plays the greater part in making you a successful communicator. The *personal* skills that win over people, both colleagues and patients, often have little to do with language. If you are 'emotionally intelligent' you are already communicating on deeper levels than spoken English can achieve through this ability to 'sense' people and how they are feeling. The need for nurses to be emotionally intelligent is being increasingly highlighted within current nursing literature (Evans and Allen 2002). You can develop your language through this emotional intelligence because both are reliant on picking up cues when listening and watching carefully. Just as you are accustomed to observing your patients carefully for 'unspoken clues', we shall be asking you to look at yourself and colleagues to pick up the finer points of communicating as a nurse.

We will also be introducing you to some other excellent resources; they will be very helpful when you want to access more information and there are more exercises to practise. In the meantime, you will be given some ideas here about how you can still work well with your patients and colleagues while your language development process at work is continuing.

What is 'UK health care English'?

As a nurse you have to communicate with many different people. On the one hand, there are medical and multidisciplinary staff such as doctors, dieticians, therapists and, of course, other nurses. At the same time, there are patients and their families. The communication with and between these different groups of people often happens in different ways, or 'registers'. This means that you use different types of language in terms of vocabulary and formality and also in attitude and perspective. Overall then, health care English in the UK is about effective communication with people according to the context in which you are placed and the needs of the people you are with.

 ## How fast can I learn?

You are not a machine. As a result, developing your confidence as you adapt to UK health care English and finding your place in your team will be a process which cannot be achieved in a day. However, you can break this process down into easy, manageable parts. These can be practical 'mini-language projects' that you carry out in the work place and, mostly, only you need to know you are doing them. These small language projects will be your exploration of how people achieve their purposes in UK health care English. That is to say, step-by-step, function-by-function, purpose-by-purpose, you can explore how and why language is being used in particular ways around you. Then you can decide which language habits you wish to mirror and use, and which you would prefer to reject! You need nothing to help you with one or two of these useful mini-projects each day but your own ability to watch and listen.

 ## What are the language challenges?

Let us focus on one of these with an observational activity which can reveal a great deal to you.

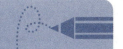

Activity

How do staff greet each other at work? How long do they spend greeting each person? Listen carefully and watch out for forms of address, body language, levels of formality and informality. Is this how you would expect to speak to a colleague?

You may be surprised that although you know and use the standard English words for greeting colleagues or friends, it sounds different when you first arrive in the work place. Remember that whenever someone speaks it is to fulfil a function, i.e. achieve a purpose. People might be using familiar words but conveying different messages. We speak, for example, to greet, persuade, get information, negotiate, apologise. You will quickly see how people at work 'manage' their relationships with each other. These will tell you about the 'power relationships' which are everywhere around you. Which people are in more 'equal' or 'friendship-based' relationships? How can you tell this from their choice of language with each other? How do we convey respect, for example?

When you have learned to notice different 'registers' amongst staff around you, turn your attention to staff/patient relationships. What do tone of voice and body language tell you? Do other staff – who may also be busy and tired – empower patients and equalise any power imbalance? Are they using different styles and registers of language as well as different body language and tone of voice?

One interesting function is 'stroking'. Briefly, stroking means saying things that make the person you are talking to feel equal, respected, valued and liked. In other words, we can think of people as being a lot like cats who will purr if you make them feel good! This idea was developed by Eric Berne in his book *Games People Play* (1964). When you are studying how people talk to each other at work, always try to notice how they 'stroke' each other – what kindnesses, compliments, helpful suggestions and support they offer. How do they thank, agree, praise, and show concern and interest? Did you notice any stroking in the greetings that you observed between staff, for example?

In any caring profession, 'stroking' is an enormously important function. In the health care setting this function is often fulfilled by the nurse's ability to **empathise**. When you 'put yourself in another person's shoes' and try for a moment to see and feel the world as they are seeing and feeling it, you are empathising. There is currently more emphasis than ever on the importance of a nurse's ability to empathise. This is regarded as essential to good nursing practice and is, in fact, a kind of emotional intelligence. In an extremely helpful book called *Hospital English, The Brilliant Learning Workbook for International Nurses* (Arakelian *et al.* 2003), this idea of using language to 'stroke' is explained very well. It is packed with useful and practical ideas or mini-projects to help you develop your 'UK health care English' in many contexts within the nurse's working environment.

But where do my English language skills come into all this?

The previous section has suggested that communication is not just about language and we will return to that theme. First, however, we want to concentrate on helping you identify where your *language* skills might needed to be practised and adapted: that is, asking a patient questions. Let's look at a task that is carried out every day in some settings – interviewing patients on admission. You would be well-advised to accompany another nurse with more experience in working in English so that you can be present during interviews. This will give you ideas about how to ask questions.

The first type is very simple direct questions. They often start with a question word such as 'What's your address?' or 'How old are you?' They can also look like this: 'Do you have any children?' These direct questions are used to collect very specific, precise and detailed information. They usually require the patient to give very brief, sometimes only 'yes/no' answers. They are also appropriate if you do not want to confuse your patient. However, if all your questions are of this type, you might appear very abrupt and unfriendly, or even aggressive. This is because, in this question type, you bring your voice down and make it sound like a statement. Therefore it is a good idea to aim for a variety of different kinds of questions in a patient interview.

The second type of question is of a much more indirect style; for instance, 'Would you mind telling me how many children you have?' or 'Could you tell me the name of your GP please?' In situations when the information you need might seem rather personal or even embarrassing to your patient, you have to ask in a much more sensitive way. Here, the indirect style question is more appropriate. At the same time, you give the patient the opportunity to say a few more words than just the specific information you want – you allow a bit of an 'open end'. Some patients might appreciate this because it gives them the feeling that you are also interested in them as people and not just patients. This type of question is often introduced by phrases such as 'Would you mind telling/showing me. . . ?' or 'Can/could you tell me. . . ?'

A third way of asking a question is to use a statement with a rising, questioning tone of voice: 'And we can contact your husband only on his mobile?' In many cases, you can start this type of question with the word 'and'. Your voice is actually extremely important and we will visit this subject later in more detail.

Activity

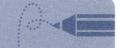

Take a blank patient admission sheet that your care setting uses. Make sure you look up any unknown or unfamiliar words in a dictionary. Then, for each of the required entries, write down at least one question you could ask. Try to use a good mix of question types, remembering which type seems most appropriate for each particular situation. Then check with a colleague and ask their advice.

When you then start interviewing, remember to introduce yourself and explain very clearly to your patient what is going to happen. Many people are quite worried about examinations in hospital or even being admitted, so it is important that you make them feel comfortable. Again, your ability to empathise is important when you explain and reassure. For example, speak to them without using abbreviations and jargon (specialist words/expressions) which the patient may not understand. Also, it is a good idea to ask the patient what he/she would like to be called and then note this down so that others in your team are aware. The way you use your body language and voice will do much to put a patient at ease and make the interview more successful. A good resource to help you with interviews and many other tasks in health care English is *Skills for Life. Effective Communication for International Nurses*, published in 2004 by the Department for Education and Skills; and which has been very helpful in the writing of this section. Much of its excellent advice and exercises can be found on the internet at **www.dfes.gov.uk/readwriteplus/embeddedlearning**.

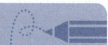

Activity

From a hospital's 'patient admission form', we have chosen the five areas below. Into each blank area, write three different questions (one of each type) you can ask the patient. The first area has been done as an example.

Example:

What the patient knows about his/her condition:

Can you tell me why you have been admitted to hospital today?

Why have you been admitted today?

And you have been admitted with suspected appendicitis?

History of present illness and reason for admission:

Relevant past medical history and medication on admission:

Allergies:

Description of home situation and accommodation:

What can I do if I'm not sure I have understood what patients are saying?

Even native speakers can misunderstand if they are not careful. Just like you, they need to check up and get clarification.

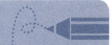
Activity

Listen carefully to how colleagues obtain clarification when they cannot be sure what a patient is saying.

Note a few of these techniques and/or questions down here. One example has already been noted for you. When you have finished, decide which seem to be the most comfortable to you and the most effective. (Adapted from Arakelian *et al.* 2003.)

Example: 'Sorry, Mrs Harding, did you say six**teen** or six**ty**?'

When you are listening carefully to how your colleagues deal with their own difficulties in understanding, notice what they do to help themselves. Their techniques will often not involve any extra words! What do they do with their voices? Do they soften them? Raise them? Lower them? What happens to their body language? Do they lean forward and look more closely at the patient?

 ## What can I do when I don't understand at all?

Why not try what we call the **'pick and repeat' technique**. When you are in difficulty understanding what people are saying, you may find it helpful to pick just one word or phrase the patient has said. Even if there are several things you could not understand properly, this technique can help you a lot further. Imagine the following interview situation:

Patient: 'Well, I was in a right two and eight at the time and went to turn round like and took a tumble. Went down like a ton of bricks.'

This patient is using a lot of colloquialisms (informal expressions): 'two and eight, turn round like, take a tumble, go down like a ton of bricks'. Actually, he is communicating almost completely here in expressions which are informal and which you might not have heard before. You cannot find out immediately what all of them mean, but you can open one door here into what the patient means by choosing, for instance, the expression 'a two and eight' so that you can **build** your under-standing of his situation around that one expression. Having targeted an unknown word or expression, repeat it back with your voice raised at the end as though the repetition was now a question.

You: 'Two and eight? Can you tell me more about that?'
Patient: 'Yeah, I was – you know, upset and getting in a panic like I do sometimes and that's how I fell again'.

Again, it is useful to remember the importance of body language. Think about how you can slow a patient down by putting your hand on theirs when you hear something you do not understand and want to get clar-ification. Eye contact is also a very valuable tool and shows your interest in detail. It is part of the language of empathy too and shows proper engagement with the patient when you are talking to them. In addition, the technique of repeating something back to a person in a questioning tone of voice that is polite and interested is something that you can use anywhere, including with other staff with whom you work.

Activity

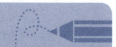

Think about how you jump easily from one register to another in your native tongue without noticing. Consider how the way you write a letter to a best friend in your native language is completely different from the way you write a job application letter or a letter of complaint to a company. What are the key differences? What would happen if you were very formal with your best friend or very informal when applying for a job?

Do make sure that you decide on a strategy – whatever it may be – so that you identify if you are having problems understanding. Imagine how frustrating it is for the speaker if you don't understand but don't say so! We would quite understand that it could be due to shyness or embarrassment, but think about the consequences. What might happen if a senior nurse passes on some vital information relating to patient care, you nod as if you understand, but it later becomes apparent that you did not understand at all? Can you imagine what that senior nurse (not to mention the patient) might think? Do remember that our placement areas are full of learners of one profession or another, and so no-one will be surprised to find you there as a language learner!

How can I get my style right?

By style you probably mean 'register'.

While you are at work you will notice that there are two or more different registers that people use. For the moment, we will concentrate on how you can often find that vocabulary is responsible for representing one register or another. Look at these:

Informal	Formal/medical
Throw up	Vomit
Feel sick	Nauseous
Be on sleeping pills	Take sedatives

You will most likely hear patients using the informal phrases on the left, often when they talk about parts of their bodies or bodily functions. Sometimes you will be able to use these too (though not always) when you are talking to your patients. Check with your colleagues which expressions are appropriate.

However, when you complete your notes and/or report back to your colleagues, try to take care to use the medical phrases on the right hand side of the table. In other words, recorded notes must be written in a more formal style. (This is important because of legal issues, which we will look at later in the section on the language of documentation.)

You will see that in your UK work place, colleagues jump registers a lot, too – without thinking about it. Often, they understand in one register and speak/write in another.

Again, do try to remember that it is not possible or necessary to record every new or unusual word or expression you meet; you might also consider getting your colleagues involved.

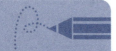

Activity

Why not choose one medical or nursing term and find out from colleagues how many different ways *they* can suggest in which patients might express this?

 ## Is pronunciation really so important?

It is not just nurses, but also doctors and other health care workers, who have problems with being understood because of their pronunciation. Remember, too, that not all of these are international workers. After all, the UK has a rich diversity of local and regional accents.

However, pronunciation can make it difficult to understand you, can lead to confusion and ambiguity, and can even sometimes cause embarrassment! For example, at a large London teaching hospital a doctor pronounced his consultant's name Hughes (quite a common English name) as if it were the word 'hugs'. It took 2 days before anyone told him the correct pronunciation (*hjooz*). When he was eventually told, he felt very embarrassed.

Nevertheless, if your communication skills as a nurse are to some extent 'hidden' by something as basic as confusing pronunciation, then some work needs to be done. It is not always possible to deal with pronunciation habits which have existed for years. But there are other ways to make yourself more easily understood.

🔑 What can I do to improve my pronunciation?

If you become aware that people have difficulty with your pronunciation, there is one simple but very effective strategy. Try to remember to speak slowly and always to face the person you are talking to so that you have as much eye contact as possible. This gives you time to check understanding by 'reading' the body language of the person with whom you are communicating. Again, this is about employing emotional intelligence to support your language and communication effectiveness. As an experienced nurse, you will most likely be good at this already.

As well as keeping eye contact as much as you can, also be aware that there are some **long vowel sounds** in English which need to be said particularly slowly. Mostly, these occur **within** words. Many overseas nurses from Africa and the Far East do not have these sounds in their own languages and for this reason find them difficult to produce. However, these sounds are important so we will look at some of them right now. There is a system of international sounds called phonemes. In any good dictionary that you are familiar with, you will see the spelling of the word you want to find but you will also find how to pronounce it. In other words, a good dictionary will also give you the word you want in phonemes so that you know how to say it. It is extremely helpful to know how to pronounce these phonemes. Here we will look at the phonemes (sounds) that tend to cause difficulties for many international nurses.

Sound /ei/

The words 'day', 'trade' and 'made' are examples of words that have the phoneme /ei/ in them. This is a long **double vowel sound**. 'Double' means that this particular phoneme actually consists of two sounds—*eh* (as in *bed*) and *ee* (as in *see*). The second sound (*ee*) often gets left out and forgotten by some speakers because they do not have these double vowel sounds in their own mother tongues. But 'day', 'trade' and 'made' are **not** pronounced *de*, *tred* or *med* but *dei*, *treid*, and *meid*. 'Day' therefore sounds like *deh-ee*. Make sure you clearly pronounce that second vowel sound, not only the first. When you listen to native speakers of English you will notice that the **second** vowel sound is very **much longer** than the first one. You will need to speak it **slowly** to produce it correctly.

Activity

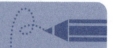

Make a list of six words that you think contain this sound. Then check in a good dictionary to see if you were right. At work, ask your mentor or someone you trust if they think you say these words correctly. If they feel you have a problem with this sound, ask them to say the words for you. Listen carefully and repeat.

Sound /ai/

This is another double vowel sound that can cause international nurses a little difficulty when they want to be understood. This is the sound in the word 'I' or 'eye'. Do you pronounce the word 'time' as *taam*? Ask a colleague if you tend to do this. If this is the case, you probably forget the **second** sound 'ee'. Again, you need to remember that the **second** sound of this double vowel sound is quite **long** and needs to be pronounced **slowly**. So the double vowel sound /ai/ is pronounced '*ah*' and '*ee*'–and 'time' sounds like *tah-eem*.

Sound /a:/

This is a long sound again, but this time it is a **single** vowel sound and sounds like a long *ah*. In good dictionaries the colon (:) after the letter is used to tell us that this is a very long sound and we must say it very slowly. If you do not do this, your versions of the words 'start' and 'heart' might sound like *stat* or *hat* and other people might find it a little difficult to understand you.

Activity

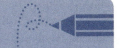

The following activity involves all three of the above-mentioned difficult sounds. Imagine that a colleague has said this to you: 'The lats were in the kapak in the dak in the ren.'

Here are the words again with some phoneme symbols to help you. Can you 'translate' this sentence into one that is now understandable?
The l/ai/ts were in the k/a:/p/a:/k in the d/a:/k in the r/ei/n.

It is important to get these sounds right. They can sometimes be a slight problem for African and Far Eastern nurses. Take great care over these **long vowel sounds** in English because, if you pronounce them too quickly, what you say may be ambiguous (have more than one meaning) and cause misunderstanding.

 ## Jargon and expressions worry me; how much can I learn on a daily basis?

Research is showing us that average language learners can learn about six new words or expressions a day – usually not more. There may be too much for you to learn immediately and you will need to accept that to learn effectively and properly you will need time.

Of course, you will meet many more than six new words or expressions a day, but two points are important. Firstly, you will need only to understand some of these but will never use them yourself. You will hear your patients or their families, and sometimes even your colleagues, use these and in the next section we will look at how you can find out what these mean. But it may not be appropriate to use them yourself, because you may appear unprofessional or even disrespectful to your patients if you do this. Thus, you will only need to understand. Secondly, many of the expressions you learn will seem to stay in your head for just a short time and then you will feel you have forgotten them. It is important to remember that this is only your perception but in reality it is not true. The new language has gone to the back of your brain. It is not lost but just 'stored', and when you meet it again you will remember that you have met it before. Research shows we often cannot learn expressions or words by hearing them or seeing them just once. We may need to meet them a few times before they are properly learned and readily available for use.

Some learners keep a small book with them – a vocabulary log – to write down the expressions they feel they must remember so that they can look at these quickly from time to time to learn them quickly and remember them. It is a very effective way to speed up the language learning process for some people and you may want to try it for a few days.

What about non-verbal communication?

As we have suggested several times already, how you say things is just as important as what you say. Take one example ... that of showing interest in the person to whom you are speaking. Most people in the UK would expect you to show interest and respect for the other person by looking them in the eye. Would you do that? Perhaps not; Ryan (2000) and Lago and Barty (2003) suggest that in some cultures it is the lack of eye-to-eye contact that conveys respect. Some people convey respect for an elder or senior by not answering but just listening, but again here that is thought of as rude. To make a 'tutting' sound between the teeth is considered usual by some people, but here in the UK it is seen as rude and unhelpful. There is an interesting tale about the acceptability of 'touching' people in Chapter 5 and that is another way of communicating that you need to consider. Many patients appreciate the empathy and support that a pat on the arm or the holding of a hand may offer, but some will not ... Look carefully at gestures such as beckoning or waving a hand in dismissal; would you use these in the same way as you see here? A colleague of ours tells a tale of a student nurse who found she had caused distress to a patient without realising, because she had not smiled! The student was performing a procedure for the first time and, in her anxiety, did not look at the patient or smile or chat ... the patient was frightened because he thought it meant something was seriously wrong with him! You might also look again at Chapter 1 on Reflective Practice, because you will need to apply those skills of self-examination in doing this. It is tempting to become 'defensive' if you feel that you have been misunderstood, but remember 'it's not *what* you do, it's *the way* that you do it!'

It is your challenge to observe the interactions of those around you and judge which behaviours appear to bring satisfaction to both parties. Those would be the behaviours that you wish to mirror.

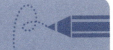

Activity

Do you feel that you or a colleague have ever been misunderstood because of cultural or other non-verbal aspects of communication? What did you do to resolve the problem?

Why is the *language* of documentation and record-keeping important?

The Nursing and Midwifery Council (NMC) provide a Code of Professional Conduct (NMC 2002a) and give very clear guidelines about documentation (NMC 2002b). Nowhere is this more important than in the writing of good care notes. These can be called as evidence when complaints are being investigated and, as Parkinson and Brooker (2004, p. 44) point out, a *'court of law will tend to assume that if care has not been recorded, then it has not been given.'* It could also be argued that the degree of professionalism or negligence the patient experienced can also be understood by a court from *the way* these records are written. If you want to read in more detail about the reasons for keeping comprehensive and accurate records, we recommend Wood's (2002) article. You probably have very similar codes or guidelines in your own country, which will help you to adapt to what is required in the UK.

The documentation you will have to provide at work is mainly for recording patient care. In many cases this involves filling in forms. There are, for instance, patient admission forms, patient assessment forms and patient care plan forms that you will have to complete on a regular basis. These forms can vary from one work place to another and each type of form will have their specific vocabulary associated with them.

Ask your manager or mentor to give you some blank copies of the different kinds of forms that your work place uses. Familiarise yourself with their layouts and language. If necessary, check words and expressions with a colleague or in a good dictionary.

Activity

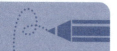

Ask your line manager or mentor whose notes you should look at as a good record-keeper. Then look at some examples of each type of completed forms (admission, assessment and care plan). For each type, note down some specific words and phrases that you have noticed are occurring more frequently than others.

No matter which of these forms you have to complete, try to involve your patients, clients or their carers whenever practicable (NMC 2002a). Always observe the following important aspects when you keep records. They are based on the two publications by the NMC mentioned above as well as the article by Wood (2002) and the Department for Education and Skills training material for international nurses (2004). Rather than provide you with an all-encompassing list we have focused on those aspects for which some practical language advice will hopefully prove useful to you.

Accuracy and objectivity

Always try and keep strictly to the facts; avoid giving your personal opinion and making speculations or judgemental statements. Subjective comments can easily give a false or distorted picture and can be offensive.

Sometimes, however, you might feel it is necessary to record your impression because it is impossible to establish a fact. To make this clear in your notes, you can use the verbs *appear* and *seem*, e.g. 'Patient *appears* to be upset' or 'Patient *seems* to be fully alert'.

When you want to record the subjective comments or impressions of a patient, introduce your comments with 'The patient/he/she said/ felt/ reported ...' and put their exact words in inverted commas; for example, 'John said that he felt "very tired and wanting to go to sleep all the time".' You can also use the expression '... as far as (Mrs X) is aware/knows ...'; for example, 'Mr Miller does not suffer from any allergies as far as he knows.'

A good way of recording information is to use so-called 'senses' verbs, e.g. 'I heard/I saw/I felt' etc., such as 'I saw a 5 cm-long cut on Mr Brown's upper arm.'

Register

In your notes, you need to use a higher level of formality than in your spoken language. As already mentioned in the section 'How can I get my style right?' you can achieve this to a great extent by choosing the right vocabulary. Use more professional medical terminology rather than generally informal, colloquial or even slang words and expressions. This is important because other health professionals will read your notes. At the same time, however, do not include jargon or overuse abbreviations; as you are aware, patients have the right to see what you are writing about them and therefore also need to be able to understand your notes. The activity part at the end of this section will explore how your sensitivity and self-discipline as an experienced, professional nurse is the **foundation** of your ability to get the vocabulary register of your written language right in your records.

Apart from the right choice of vocabulary, you can use another language feature to make your writing more formal. You achieve this by focusing more on the patient and the procedures rather than on reporting what you (or the doctor) do/did. This feature is called 'passive voice' (in contrast to 'active voice'). Here are two examples. Instead of writing 'I took the patient to the X-ray department,' you might prefer to record 'Patient was taken to X-ray department.' Instead of 'I have given patient a new pair of TED stockings', you might write 'patient was given new pair of TED stockings'.

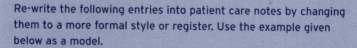

Activity

Re-write the following entries into patient care notes by changing them to a more formal style or register. Use the example given below as a model.

Rather than writing 'I monitored the blood pressure every 15 minutes for 2 hours after the operation,' write 'Blood pressure was monitored every 15 minutes for 2 hours after the operation.'

Active voice (slightly informal)	Passive voice (slightly more formal)
The GP prescribed several courses of antibiotics	
I informed the patient of the reasons for and consequences of the procedures	
I administered the prescribed nebuliser at 2-hourly intervals	

Avoid ambiguity

In your notes, take great care not to use language that could have different meanings to different people. If your colleagues do not know what you mean, your notes will become at best meaningless, and at worst, can lead to confusion, misunderstanding or misinterpretation. For example, if you write '. . . with large bruises on his back . . .,' the word *large* in this case could describe for you an area of 3 cm diameter whereas your supervisor would not have considered this to be *large*. Another example is the abbreviation PT which can stand for patient, physiotherapist or part time (Wood 2002). In many cases, it is adjectives and adverbs, but also abbreviations, that can cause ambiguity. Many areas will have lists of agreed or standardised expressions that are known to all staff. If this is the case, make sure that you use them. If they are not available, why not try to compile one with your colleagues?

Always try to be as precise as possible. Instead of ambiguous adjectives and adverbs, use clear and precise expressions. For example, instead of *early/late* or other general time words, use the exact time, such as 8 am or 10 pm. Instead of general words such as *good* or *well*, e.g. 'patient had a good day' or 'patient slept well', describe exactly what you mean by using less ambiguous expressions such as 'patient was pleased to have visitors and appeared to be cheerful for the rest of the day' or 'patient reported undisturbed sleep.'

Relevance and clarity

In your notes, record only details and information that is relevant to the treatment or care of the patient at that time. If you or other staff have to read through lengthy notes that do not provide vital, important information this might waste a lot of time which you could spend more effectively on other activities. Equally dangerous are very long sentences without full stops. They can confuse many points and important information might not be recorded properly or missed out completely. Therefore good records are generally not written in long, complete sentences but in note form. However, they must still include all the relevant and important points and be clear and precise for other staff to understand them.

Try to make your sentences short and clear. To write in note form, you can often leave out 'little' words that are not essential. These are typically words such as articles (*the*, *a/an*), auxiliary verbs (is, are, has, have) and pronouns (he, she) or even the patient's name (as long as it is obvious whose notes they are!). On the other hand, you must include words that are necessary to get the important information across; that means words that carry a lot of meaning. These words are usually nouns, verbs, adjectives, adverbs, numerals and frequently prepositions.

Compare the following complete sentences with the note form entries. Check if the nurse who wrote the notes has followed the advice given above. Pay special attention to how negative sentences change. Note any other changes that have taken place. (This activity has been slightly adapted from DfeS 2004 *Skills for Life*: p. 87).

Full sentences	Note form entries
He was admitted to hospital 2 days ago and he had a terrible pain in his chest.	Admitted to hospital 2 days ago with severe chest pain
She said that she had felt very weak yesterday and then she actually passed out while she was shopping with her daughter.	Felt very weak yesterday and lost consciousness whilst out shopping
As far as Mr Jones is aware, he has never had any problems with his digestion.	No history of digestive problems
She says she isn't allergic to any foods.	No known food allergies

Activity

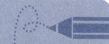

Now have a go yourself. Change the following extracts into note form. Then check your suggestions with a colleague or mentor.

Full sentences	Note form entries
Mrs Brooks has never been in hospital before and is really anxious about what might happen to her because her husband died in the same hospital a year ago.	
She and her husband never had a car and she walks to the local shops every other day. She says she is so pleased that she can still do everything by herself – so many people of her age need some help from their families or neighbours.	
Recently she has gone off her food. She cooks all the meals she and her husband used to like but she simply doesn't feel like eating anything at all.	

Do remember that there are plenty of other exercises to practise in the resources that we have recommended, and the more you try, the easier it will become.

Summary

In summary, this chapter has covered a great deal of valuable
information that has enabled you to:
- ✔ Discuss the importance of communication for nurses.
- ✔ Reflect on some cultural and non-verbal aspects of communication.
- ✔ Identify key language challenges for nursing in the UK.
- ✔ Consider your own language development needs.
- ✔ Decide how you will meet some of these needs.

References

Arakelian C, Bertram C and Magnall A (2003). *Hospital English. The Brilliant Learning Workbook for International Nurses*. London: Penguin.

Berne E (1964). *Games People Play*. London: Andre Deutsche.

Department for Education and Skills (2004). *Skills for Life. Effective Communication for International Nurses. Materials for Embedded Learning*. London: DfES.

Evans D and Allen H (2002). Emotional intelligence: its role in training. *Nursing Times* **98(27)**: 41–42. Retrieved from http://www.nursingtimes.net

Lago C and Barty A (2003). *Working with International Students : Cross-cultural Training Manual*. London: UKCOSA.

Nursing and Midwifery Council (2002a). *The Code of Professional Conduct*. London: NMC.

Nursing and Midwifery Council (2002b). *Guidelines for Records and Record Keeping*. London: NMC.

Parkinson J and Brooker C (2004). *Everyday English for International Nurses: A Guide to Working in the UK*. Edinburgh: Churchill Livingstone.

Ryan J (2000). *A Guide to Teaching International Students*. Oxford: Oxonian Press.

Wood C (2002). The importance of good record-keeping for nurses. *Nursing Times* **99(2)**: 26–27.

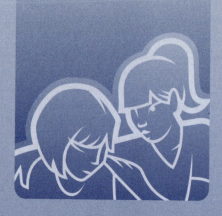

Chapter 7

What does the future hold for you as a nurse in the UK?

David Maher

This chapter will look to the future – yours and that of nursing and care services in the UK. The chapter will enable you to:

✔ Identify how professionals keep knowledge and skills up to date
✔ Look at the range of post-qualifying education that is available to you
✔ Explore specialist roles that are developing in nursing
✔ Consider recent and future changes to nursing and health care that may affect you
✔ Set some goals and plan your future!

Having registered with the Nursing and Midwifery Council (NMC) many nurses stay for a period of time to consolidate their experience and gain skills which they intend eventually to take back to their home country, or elsewhere. For others, the UK becomes their home and many people settle here indefinitely and wish to develop their careers in what is a challenging yet rewarding environment. Some nurses may decide that nursing in the UK is not for them and return home for a variety of reasons, including homesickness, financial pressures and family priorities. It is hoped that, by the end of the chapter, you will feel able to participate in the many continuing professional development opportunities that are available to you, and feel a valued and respected member of the health care team wherever your chosen career takes you.

 ## What are the changing roles and responsibilities in the UK?

In the UK, the first groups of people to be defined as a profession were involved in the law, the church and medicine (Phillips 2004). Clearly, it is impossible to outline the cultural, social and political history of professional development in this chapter but, to help you understand the context of professionalism in the UK, the **traditional characteristics of a profession** are listed below:

- A duty of public care and service
- A unique body of knowledge associated with professional practice
- A prescribed period of education (defined as 5 years)
- Controlled entry and standards of practice
- A professional body regulated by law with disciplinary powers
- A code of conduct
- Autonomous practice

(Etzioni 1969, Brook 1974)

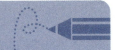

Activity

How is a professional defined in your country?

Which health care workers in your country are regarded as professionals?

Ask colleagues who you currently work with in the UK who they regard as professionals. What differences and similarities are there between your country and the UK?

In the UK, there is still some debate as to whether nursing can be regarded as a true profession as its body of knowledge is often drawn from many other areas, including psychology, medicine and the natural sciences, making its uniqueness questionable (Colyer 2004, Phillips 2004). Alternatively, the application of this knowledge by nurses could be regarded as unique as they address the social, physical, psychological and spiritual needs of patients in a holistic manner (Gustafsson and Fagerberg 2004). Whilst nursing work is often interdependent on other professionals (such as doctors and social workers), and their work is never truly autonomous, it could be argued that this applies to all health professionals, who rely on mutual understanding and agreement to practise effectively. As health needs become more complex, it is likely that no single professional can hope to have the necessary skills and knowledge to care for patients autonomously and, as such, old definitions such as those outlined previously in this chapter are becoming redundant (Huotari 2003, Integrated Care Network 2004).

Phillips (2004) suggests that 'the essence of professionalism is to be able to call upon the honour, probity and principled judgement of the practitioner' and, to this end, it would appear that it is the characteristics of the individual rather than the professional knowledge and skills of groups of people that is significant. This is an important point to bear in mind as you start your career in the UK, as professional identities and roles are changing and new ways of working are becoming more common. Increasingly, nurses are working as part of a wider team and taking on additional duties and responsibilities to reflect their skills which are very different from the traditional role of the nurse. Similarly, as health and social care organisations realise the potential advantage of working more closely together, you may find that you work with colleagues from other organisations, which requires clear leadership and effective management skills (Integrated Care Network 2004, DoH 2005).

 ## How is government policy supporting change?

Clinical governance represents one of the biggest policy shifts in the NHS in recent times, and it is essential for you to have some understanding of its relevance to you. Clinical governance requires that organisations within the NHS attempt to evaluate not only professional practice, but review and change the way the organisation is run to ensure it maximises benefit to patients (Vanu Som 2004). This may involve reviewing budgetary arrangements, the use of physical space and changing traditional routines as well as ensuring that human resources such as doctors, nurses and physiotherapists are available in sufficient numbers with the right level of skill to meet patient need.

Another aim of clinical governance is to ensure that professionals have the necessary skills to retrieve and understand research and other evidence to develop their knowledge and skills for practice (DoH 1998). This has challenged many nurses as they realised that what they used to do when performing patient care was often based on tradition and customs rather than evidence.

Whilst professionals have always attempted to ensure care is of high quality, there was very little consistency in how this was done across the country, and many patients and professionals complained that a 'post code lottery' existed whereby the quality and availability of care offered depended upon where you lived (DoH 1999). In addition to the clinical governance framework, a great deal of government policy has sought to tackle some of the major weaknesses of the NHS. These are outlined in Table 7.1 and expanded upon in Chapter 3.

Table 7.1 Key policy themes and priorities

- Inequality – poorer people were likely to die younger, have more preventable illnesses and access health care resources less frequently
- Higher rates of death in the UK from preventable causes such as coronary heart disease, cancer and mental health problems compared to other developed countries
- Delays with diagnosing and treating illnesses throughout the NHS because of resource deficits, lack of integrated planning and working between professionals and managers
- Ensuring care is delivered that meets patient needs and is evaluated by patients at all levels

In an attempt to rectify this situation, clinical governance should be regarded as the means through which government can drive through its many health policies (Vanu Som 2004). It is often a major influence on how local Trusts operate and prioritise their activities to ensure care offered is of high quality and meets government set targets. You will come across a range of activities and practices that fall into the clinical governance framework. The most common of these are outlined in Table 7.2.

Table 7.2 Activities associated with clinical governance

Activity /focus	Examples
Clinical audit	Where professionals measure local performance against a set standard which reflects research. Examples include case review, benchmarking and peer review
Risk management	Strategies in place to ensure each organisation and professional assesses potential risk of patient harm and takes appropriate measures to eliminate or manage unavoidable risk
Clinical guideline development groups	To ensure that local guidelines reflect best practice as defined in research – often assisted by institutions such as NICE (National Institute of Health and Clinical Excellence)
Workforce planning and development	Trusts and Strategic Health Authorities must identify future health needs of the local population and secure appropriate education and training to ensure that needs are met by professionals with the right level of knowledge and skills
Identifying clear lines or responsibilities in professional and organisational structures	For example, the development of single assessment policies, integrated care pathways, user involvement groups

It is in this context that the changes in roles and professional responsibilities need to be viewed and understood so that you can make sense
of what you may experience and appreciate how to make the most of
the personal and professional opportunities that clinical governance
and other policy initiatives offer now and in the future. Education and
training to develop hands-on care skills are still important, but many
nurses find themselves needing to develop different skills and knowledge to reflect some of the activities and priorities listed above to
enable them to enhance their careers.

Activity

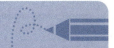

Are you familiar with any of the activities listed, such as risk
management or clinical audit?

What benefits do you think they might offer to health services?

 **How do I maintain registration as a
nurse?**

The NMC was established by an Act of Parliament to regulate nursing
and midwifery practice and standards, and to maintain a live register of
all practitioners. It is also responsible for offering advice on professional standards and for considering allegations of misconduct. Its
main aim, therefore, should be seen as protecting the public. To achieve
this aim, the NMC developed a framework for professional development
known as PREP (Post Registration Education and Practice; NMC 2004).

PREP stipulates that all registered nurses and midwives must renew
their registration every 3 years to continue to practise (NMC 2004). As
part of the renewal process, you will be required to confirm that you
have met the standards set out in Table 7.3.

Table 7.3 NMC PREP standards

The NMC requires that each nurse or midwife:

- Has worked for a minimum of 450 hours in a capacity that required a nursing or midwifery qualification, or completed an approved return to practise course in the previous 3 years prior to renewal. For practitioners with dual qualifications, for example in nursing and midwifery, this standard applies to each qualification.
- Undertakes a minimum of 35 hours' learning activities that are relevant to his/her practice during the 3 years prior to renewal.
- Maintains a record of all continuing professional development activities undertaken in the previous 3 years prior to renewal in the form of a personal professional portfolio.
- Complies with any NMC request to audit their professional development portfolio.

 ## What is personal development planning?

You will gain experience of developing personal development plans during your preparation for registration, although you may view it as 'goal setting'. Once qualified, such plans allow you and your employer to negotiate mutually beneficial activities and training in a planned and systematic way. Often, training need is identified as a result of your performance review (appraisal) and personal career ambitions, and it is a good idea to consider these in advance of any meeting with your preceptor, mentor or manager, perhaps logging your thoughts in a reflective diary or even in your professional portfolio so that you are well prepared. The following exercise may help you prepare well to negotiate study and training support, either during your ONP or afterwards.

Activity

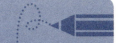

Think through the following questions as if you were proposing a course for yourself ...

- What priorities has your manager/organisation set for your area of practice?
- How will your chosen study/training session help to improve care of patients or families in your area of practice; how do these relate to the organisational goals?
- What do you need and what are you willing to contribute in order to undertake this training (funding, study time)?
- How will you ensure that your new skills/knowledge are effectively disseminated to colleagues?

 ## What kind of education and training is available for qualified nurses?

During the course of your career in the UK, you will be exposed to many different learning experiences, some of which will be formal (perhaps at a university), whilst others may be from practice or as a result of your reflective skills. Learning is often stimulating and rewarding, but can also be associated with a degree of discomfort as existing knowledge is tested and attitudes challenged (Pross 2005). This may be particularly true for you as you progress in your career as you will come across care practices that seem to be alien or 'wrong', or which challenge your sense of what nursing is about (RCN 2003). The good news is that you will not be alone, as most nurses feel this way at some point in their career and may be willing to offer support and alternative interpretations of a given situation. Perhaps the best way of looking at learning is to think of it as a chance to discover and understand more about yourself, your practice, the patient and his/her family, as this will almost certainly help you to manage the many challenges that being a nurse brings.

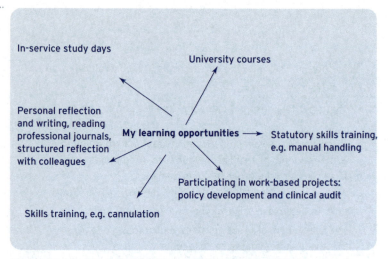

Figure 7.1 Learning opportunities available to the qualified nurse

Deciding how to plan your professional development can be difficult as you will be stimulated by different things at different times and, often, your original thoughts will change with experience and exposure to new opportunities and challenges posed by patients, your manager and the organisation as a whole. For this reason, it is crucial that you take time to work with your mentor, preceptor and manager to create a personal development plan that works for you and everyone else concerned.

Studying at university

Many nurses complete university-based learning as it enables you to explore new ways of working safely and develop knowledge relating to a specific subject that is reliably and rigorously assessed through the completion of assignments and/or examinations set by qualified teachers. Whilst you will have completed assignments during your preparation for registration, you may need to consider how easily you will cope with formal written English, even if you scored well in your IELTS. The type of writing you do for work or pleasure is quite different from the type of writing required in an essay, for example. Similarly, set assignments, such as essays or case studies, may be very different in the UK to those with which you are familiar in your home country. These challenges can be overcome by finding out what support is available within the university, as well as accessing the wide range of support offered by local further education colleges or skills training centres. Alternatively, there is a range of internet-based learning packages available that will help you to differentiate between a comma and a semi-colon, not to mention where to place an apostrophe!

Whilst individual courses may be valuable to you and your practice, many can be studied together to contribute to a formal academic award such as a degree or postgraduate award. Increasingly, promotion is dependent on experience as well as the acquisition of formal academic qualifications. In Chapter 6, you have read that the English language is often confusing and 'strange', and therefore you are strongly advised to clarify any questions about your study with the tutor responsible for admissions to make sure that you enrol onto the correct module to meet your needs and determine the right level of study in your particular circumstance.

University-based learning uses a variety of methods to teach in addition to traditional class-based learning. Some offer a range of learning packages that can be studied from a distance (distance learning). Others utilise the internet and information technology to offer class-based, work-based and 'virtual' learning in combination; this is often referred to as 'blended' learning. It is important to consider what your personal learning preferences are so that if, for example, you like to learn in group settings and enjoy debate and discussion on a regular basis, distance learning may not be the right choice for you as it involves a lot of self-directed study on your own.

Strategic Health Authorities allocate a budget for training and education which is managed by local NHS Trusts. This money is available for nurses, but competition is high and it is often targeted at training and education that enables the organisation involved to meet its needs. It may be possible to obtain support with funding from a variety of other sources, such as charitable organisations and drug companies. However, many nurses fund themselves to advance their career and to select an education that meets their personal interests. Self-funding is often regarded as an investment, and many universities offer a variety of payment methods to ease the financial burden.

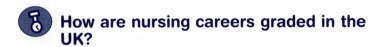 ## How are nursing careers graded in the UK?

It is likely that once you gain some experience you will want to think about your career direction and, to do this, you need to be aware of the vast range of jobs and roles that nurses perform in the UK, and the qualifications and skills that are required to fulfil them.

The NHS is Europe's largest employer (**www.nhscareers.nhs.uk**) and nurses play a role in almost every part of it. Until recently most nurses involved in caring for patients were graded from bands C to I. Generally speaking, skills, experience and responsibilities as well as salary increased as you progressed towards grade I. In 2004, a new grading system was introduced as a result of a Department of Health review known as Agenda for Change (DoH 2004a). This aims to link salary to the application of skills and knowledge required to fulfil a particular role, and is linked closely to the Knowledge and Skills Framework (KSF) (DoH 2004b). There are six core domains associated with the KSF which are applicable to all health workers, and 24 specific domains, some of which may not be appropriate for some groups (for example, estates and facilities is a specific domain which most nurses would not be working to, whereas health and well being is very relevant to nurses). These 30 domains are divided into four different levels of working, representing more complex roles and functions. The idea is that as you improve your knowledge and skills in your role, you will work at a higher level of responsibility and have different expectations placed upon you than someone working at a lower level of skill, and therefore you should be eligible for a different salary band. It is too soon to determine whether this new framework will be effective but it is likely that the KSF will be a major influence on your professional development, and you are likely to want to study courses and gain specific skills that reflect the areas outlined in the KSF. You can find out more about Agenda for Change and the Knowledge Skills Framework by visiting the Department of Health website (**www.doh.gov.uk**).

What about working in specialist roles?

Most newly registered nurses will work in health settings such as a hospital ward, community or nursing home, performing direct patient care duties. This is an important time as it allows you to experience caring for a diverse range of patients with different illnesses and conditions so that you can consolidate your knowledge and skills and adjust to the responsibilities of being a registered nurse in the UK. During the first year or two, it is likely that this 'settling in' period will be associated with learning 'on the job' and establishing yourself as a team member. Some people decide that they like the variety of general nursing and opt to remain in general environments throughout their career, whether in direct patient care roles, managerial roles or specialist areas of responsibility such as risk management. Other nurses decide that they want to develop skills in a specialist area of practice, whether in NHS hospitals, the independent sector, commercial companies or community-based organisations. The range of options available to you is very broad and, as 'Arthur's' case below demonstrates, nursing can involve caring in many different ways and in various locations, using different levels of skill and knowledge. To understand some of this activity, we shall look at Arthur and identify the nurse involved in his care in varying roles, and then look at the work of Kate, who is a specialist nurse.

Case Study

'Arthur' is a 65-year-old man admitted to hospital 2 weeks ago with a myocardial infarction (MI). He phoned NHS Direct (a health information helpline manned by nurses 24 hours a day, 7 days a week) and sought advice from the nurse advisor, which led him to call an ambulance. In the accident and emergency department, he was assessed by the emergency nurse practitioner and taken to the coronary care unit where he was cared for by a team of nurses who specialise in coronary care. Jo works in the unit, is recently qualified and has no specific qualifications; her colleague Nisha has just completed a post-registration module at a university and gained promotion as a team leader. The ward sister has a degree in critical care nursing and is currently studying an MSc in health management. When he was ready for discharge, Arthur was introduced to the cardiac rehabilitation team and met Hamid, one of the nurses who has specialised in helping patients live well after an MI. Arthur experienced considerable problems with his health immediately after his discharge home and was assessed by the district nurses and hospital-based nurse consultant. Eventually, Arthur recovered fully and was able to live an independent life, free of nurses apart from his wife, who is a former nurse!

That was a look at nursing roles from the patient's perspective, but now let us look at the nurse: Kate is a nurse with many years' experience who took a career break when her children were small and has relatively recently returned to nursing. She now works as a nurse practitioner in a genitourinary medicine clinic. This is how Kate describes her work:

I see my own patients, either referred from GPs or 'open access' referrals. The latter are patients who decide for themselves that they wish to be seen in clinic. I take a history, do a full physical examination, and arrange the blood tests and any other investigations that are needed. I also perform a risk assessment, which is very important with this group of patients. Once I have made a diagnosis, I prescribe treatment using patient group directives, but when I have completed the non-medical prescribing course, I will be prescribing on my own. I also carry out some of the treatments such as cryotherapy. I would say that you have to be decisive and able to take responsibility, but above all, in this job, you need wonderful communication skills so that you can support people who may be feeling vulnerable or embarrassed.

One of the difficulties that you may encounter as you progress in your career is the lack of clarity as to what a specialist nursing role actually involves in terms of competence and knowledge. There is a multitude of job titles and roles that nurses perform but, with the exception of community specialist practitioners, there is no standard of post-qualification practice recordable with the NMC (NMC 2005) and therefore monitoring performance is impossible. This causes some confusion for patients and their families as well as for health care teams, who have no common expectation of what specialist nurses actually do and the level of competence that they have.

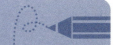

Activity

What did you think of these two descriptions of nursing roles?

What does the term 'specialist nurse' mean to you? Compare your thoughts with others in your team, including any specialist nurses with whom you come into contact.

What is clear is that a specialist nurse can be thought of in terms of the role he/she fulfils and that they often have experience and qualifications in a given area of practice above that required of most other nurses. Most specialist nurses tend to manage a caseload, make a differential diagnosis, manage care and treatment in conjunction with others, and offer leadership, support and advice to the wider health care team (NMC 2005). By using this expertise, specialist nurses are often able to resolve difficulties in complex cases and situations. The NMC entered into a period of consultation with the profession relating to recording post-qualifying practice standards which ended in February 2005 but, as yet, no standard has been published. There is considerable controversy about this and many nurses who are currently employed as specialist nurses may or may not have the necessary skills, knowledge and competence to fulfil any newly defined standard.

By entering into a specialist area of practice or developing specific skills based on interest, the nurse can gain experience and develop knowledge and skills at variable levels of ability which may or may not lead to a specialist level of practice or role. Quite often, nurses enter into a specialist area of practice and find that the reality is very different from their initial perception. There is a big difference in occasionally doing something and doing it all the time and, for this reason, it is best to consider the advantages and disadvantages of specialising carefully and perhaps arrange a period of time working in a specific environment or shadowing a specialist role holder. This is an example of how professional development planning can really help you to explore different options and opportunities.

 ## What other changes are likely?

Nursing has changed enormously since the days of Florence Nightingale but at its heart remains the concern for people and care delivery. It is likely that, over the next 10 or 20 years, health and nursing care will go through several more changes as new knowledge is discovered and new ways of working are implemented as a result of government policy. To cope well with this and to ensure that your voice is heard, you will need to understand what is happening around you. This is why continuing professional development is a compulsory part of being a professional and is such an important part of UK nursing. By keeping up to date with best practice and research and acquiring new skills, you will be able to make a better contribution to patient care no matter which role you perform at what grade. This will enhance your self-esteem and confidence, and the result will be a rich and rewarding career that benefits you, the patients you care for, the organisation that you work in, and humanity as a whole.

As technology and science continue to unravel some of the mysteries of illness and disease, it is likely that health care professionals will face increasing difficulty in applying this potential in their practice. Increasingly, the scope of science and technology to affect human life, health and death is enormous, and it raises many questions relating to what is right and proper and where the scope or boundary of innovation should be drawn. Such innovation is difficult as it raises moral and ethical issues that are likely to challenge the government, health services, professionals and individuals alike as they try to decide what is and is not acceptable and how the advantages of new innovation will be distributed across the population fairly. It is also likely that health care costs will continue to spiral upwards and force the country to examine its priorities and balance health needs with other areas of expenditure such as education, defence and transport. This will cause inevitable debate and possible tension between individuals, organisations and the state as well as wider international communities as health becomes a major factor in international relationships and disputes (Kirk 2002).

In relation to the UK, the application of new scientific discoveries and technologies is likely to change the way in which health care is delivered, understood and organised. Outlined below are some of the issues that are emerging, with suggestions of others that may develop in the future. You may be able to add some of your own.

Potential health challenges and benefits

- Establishing the best system in which to deliver health care – state run, social insurance schemes, private companies
- The cost of sustaining an ageing population – financial, social and moral
- Increase in the incidence of chronic illnesses such as heart disease, cancer, diabetes, neurological illnesses and mental illness, owing to age and occupational causes
- Less clear 'responsibility' or 'duty' to care for ageing relatives as family structures continue to change – divorce, step-children, geographically dispersed families
- Illness prevention legislation – individual freedom and choice versus public health relating to smoking, obesity and sexual behaviours, for example
- Ensuring new treatments are equally distributed irrespective of age, class, gender, race, etc.
- Rationing – criteria used. Is it made explicit who decides: government, public or professionals?
- Is it right to keep people alive at all costs, let them die naturally, or end their life through assisted death?
- Coping with diverse opinion, beliefs and moral stances – liberty and oppression of exploration
- Longer 'healthier' life for most of the population

➤

- Greater productivity from a healthier population able to work longer and pay for any increase in the cost of health care
- Eradication/better management of diseases such as cancer, diabetes, AIDS, dementia, etc. arising out of new and better treatments/preventative measures
- Potential reduction in chronic disease incidence and impact on quality of life owing to medical advancement, therefore reduced financial and social burden to society

Activity

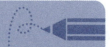

What health-related technological and scientific innovations are you familiar with in your home country and how do these compare to what is happening in the UK?

Consider some of the benefits and difficulties such discoveries may bring.

What is certain is that in order to meet these challenges and maximise the potential of such technologies, nurses will need to develop new skills and knowledge whether in research, delivering care, managing care and organisations, or educating the workforce. To do this it is important to examine what a professional actually is and the responsibilities placed on nurses to maintain and update their skills and knowledge.

Summary

This chapter has considered:

✔ Recent policy developments such as clinical governance and KSFs.
✔ The importance of personal development planning and continuing professional education.
✔ The opportunities available for post-qualification education.
✔ Specialist roles in nursing.
✔ Some future challenges for you and nursing in the UK.

References

Brook D (1974). *Education for the Professions*. London: Macmillan.

Colyer H (2004). The construction and development of health professions: where will it end? *Journal of Advanced Nursing* **48(4)**: 406-412.

DoH (1998). *A First-Class Service: Quality in the New NHS*. London: Department of Health.

DoH (1999). *Saving Lives: Our Healthier Nation*. London: Department of Health.

DoH (2004a). *Agenda For Change*. London: Department of Health.

DoH (2004b). *The NHS Knowledge and Skills Framework (NHS KSF) and the Development of Review Process*. London: Department of Health.

DoH (2005). *Delivering a Patient-led NHS*. London: Department of Health.

Etzioni A (1969). *The Semi-professions and their Organisation*. New York: Free Press.

Gustafsson C and Fagerberg I (2004). Reflection, the way to professional development? *Journal of Clinical Nursing* **13**: 271-280.

Huotari R (2003). Contradictions in interprofessional care: possibilities for change and development. *Journal of Interprofessional Care* **17(2)**: 151-160.

Integrated Care Network (2004). *Integrated Working: a Guide*. **www.integratedcarenetwork.org.uk**

Kirk M (2002). The impact of globalization and environmental change on health: challenges for nurse education. *Nurse Education Today* **22(1)**: 60-71.

NMC (2004). *The PREP Handbook*. London: Nursing and Midwifery Council.

NMC (2005). *Consultation on a Framework for the Standard for Post-registration Nursing*. London: Nursing and Midwifery Council.

Phillips A (2004). Are the liberal professions dead and if so, does it matter? *Clinical Medicine* **4**: 7-9.

Pross E (2005). International nursing students: a phenomenological perspective. *Nurse Education Today* **25**: 627-633.

RCN (2003). *'We Need Respect' Experiences of Internationally Recruited Nurses in the UK*. London: Royal College of Nursing.

Vanu Som C (2004). Clinical governance: a fresh look at its definition. *Clinical Governance: An International Journal* **9(2)**: 87-90.

www.nhscareers.nhs.uk/aboutnhs.ntml accessed 2 May 2006.

Glossary

AEI – Approved Educational Institution or Higher Education Institution (HEI) University approved by the NMC to offer programmes that lead to NMC registration.

AfC – Agenda for Change A new pay and reward system which aims to provide equal pay for work of equal value for all NHS staff. It also hopes to provide a career framework for staff to develop within their present roles and to prepare them for new roles.

AHP – Allied Health Professional Professionals such as physiotherapists, paramedics and radiographers who work alongside medical and nursing colleagues. Regulated by the Health Professions Council.

BBC – British Broadcasting Company Public service broadcasters on TV and Radio, also at http://www.bbc.co.uk

Clinical governance The national framework intended to render NHS organisations accountable for continuously improving the quality of their services and safeguarding high standards of care.

DfES – Department for Education and Skills Government department with overall responsibility for policy and services relating to education and training in the UK.

DH – Department of Health Government department with overall responsibility for policy and services relating to health and social care in the UK.

EU – European Union European Economic Community (EEC) countries and states of Europe bound by common laws and mutual agreements such as freedom of movement to work and travel.

GP – General Practitioner Medical doctor who works in the community or 'primary care', often called the 'family doctor'.

ICS – Independent Care Sector Care providers who operate outside the public funding of the NHS, and include both business and non-profit organisations, also called 'private sector'.

IELTS – International English Language Testing System Testing method chosen by the NMC to determine language proficiency for overseas applicants.

KSF – Knowledge and Skills Framework Overarching framework of knowledge and skills for all health care workers, organised into core and disciplinary domains. The four levels of working represent progress to advanced or more complex roles.

NHS – National Health Service Nationwide system of provision of care and treatment for all age groups, free at the point of use.

NICE – National Institute for Clinical Excellence NICE is an NHS organisation responsible for providing national guidance and guidelines on promoting good health and preventing and treating ill-health.

NMC – Nursing and Midwifery Council Regulatory body for nurses and midwives in the four countries of the UK.

NSFS – National Service Frameworks Long-term strategies for improving specific areas of care. They set national standards and identify key interventions for a defined service or care group.

PCT – Primary Care Trust NHS trust responsible for providing community-based services and commissioning hospital care and services.

PREP – Post Registration Education and Practice NMC framework to guide professional development and facilitate periodic re-registration. Details at http://www.nmc-org.uk

RCN – Royal College of Nursing Professional and trades union for nurses. Details at http://www.rcn.org.uk

Registrant Nurse or midwife registered as a practising professional with the NMC.

SHA – Strategic Health Authority Bodies that manage and fund the NHS at local level and are accountable to the Department of Health.

UNISON Trades union for nurses and health care workers. Details at http://www.unison.org.uk

Index